LIVING WITH A COLOSTOMY

Based on many years' experience as a colostomist, the
author gives sound, practical advice on coping with the day-
to-day problems involved in colostomy living.

LIVING WITH
A COLOSTOMY
practical advice on overcoming the problems

by

MARGARET SCHINDLER

TURNSTONE
TURNSTONE PRESS LIMITED
Wellingborough, Northamptonshire

This revised edition first published 1985

British Library Cataloguing in Publication Data

Schindler, Margaret
  Living with a colostomy: reassuring advice on
  returning to normal life after a colostomy
  operation. — Rev. ed.
  1. Colostomy
  I. Title
  362.1'975547   RD543.C6

ISBN 0-85500-222-0

*Turnstone Press is part of the
Thorsons Publishing Group*

Printed and bound in Great Britain

ACKNOWLEDGEMENTS

Mr Arthur C. Akehurst, FRCS, Consultant Surgeon. Emily Brain, MBE, General Secretary, Colostomy Welfare Group (Rtd). Jill Catto, Stoma Care Nurse, RSCN, RGN. Megan Palmer, County Organizer Home Help Service (Rtd). Air Commodore A. James Ronald, CBE, AFC, MA(Oxon), Welfare Officer. Joan M. Short, Senior Nursing Officer, Education/Community. M. R. Thomas, Nursing Officer, Community. Phyllis Turner, Welfare Officer. And all those Ostomists and relatives who have been so helpful with Surveys and Interviews. Finally all Consultants, surgeons, nursing staffs, Community Nurses and GPs who have always been ready to advise.

And Dr F. Tennant Schindler, helpmate, checkmate, and playmate.

CONTENTS

PREFACE

This book is not meant to be a medical treatise on the care and management of a colostomy or stoma. I hope it will prove to be a simple statement of various ideas, problems and possible solutions which may occur after the patient has returned home from hospital and is without the caring attention of surgeons and nurses. Basically it will look at how ordinary people endeavour to cope, for we are all novices when it comes to the actual management of a new life.

Therefore, these are an ostomist's observations and experiences over more than twenty-three years of living with a stoma. If any one of the observations included here is of help to one person (be it a colostomist, ileostomist, relative, stoma-care nurse or the community nurse who will now have the after-care nursing responsibility), it will have been more than worthwhile.

I have used the word 'patient' sparingly as the object of this book is to regard well-recovered colostomists and ileostomists physically, mentally and sexually healthy people, albeit a little different in their physical image.

INTRODUCTION

There are two operations resulting in a stoma (an opening) for the disposal of the waste matter from the body, and below I give a broad definition of each.

Colostomy. This operation is performed when there is an obstruction or disease in the bowel, necessitating the removal of the rectum and the diseased part of the colon, hence the word 'colostomy'.

An opening is made in the abdominal wall, usually on the lower left side above the hip bone. The siting of the opening is very carefully worked out by the surgeon, according to the weight, fatty tissue, and of course, the condition of the patient. Sometimes the stoma is placed higher in the abdominal wall.

The healthy bowel is joined to the stoma, and the waste matter from the bowel is then passed into a disposable plastic bag or dressing.

Patients with a colostomy are usually middle-aged, the ratio between men and women being about equal.

Ileostomy. This operation is commonly performed when there has been much pain and diarrhoea, and necessitates the large intestine being by-passed, bringing the ileum to a stoma opening, hence the word 'ileostomy'. This stoma is usually sited higher up on the right-hand side.

The reasons for this operation are often different from the colostomy, the patient usually being under forty years of age. The care of an ileostomy is also different from that of a colostomy as the waste matter is looser, because more of the intestine has been removed or diverted at an earlier stage of the disposal process.

In most patients the waste has to be eliminated through a 'disposable' plastic open-ended bag.

Statistically, more women than men have this operation.

There are an estimated 200,000 colostomists and ileostomists in Britain, with some 7,000 operations being performed every year, some being temporary, others being permanent. It is not known exactly how many there are, as for many years proper records were not kept. Also, many patients, once the operation had been performed, did not wish their stoma to be known, so repeated visits to the hospitals, and more recently, the Stoma Clinics, were difficult to maintain and assess.

I hope this book is going to bring to the fore ideas and methods so that colostomists may return to a fuller and happier life.

As a bonus, it may also give ileostomists some useful hints. I know as a vintage colostomist, that private chats I have had with ileostomists have been definitely helpful to them.

The first indication that something is not right can take several forms, and may at first be ignored as a passing condition. Often patients feel that the operation has taken them unawares, as there has been no apparent signs of trouble, but upon reflection there could have been indications which may have suggested a visit to the General Practitioner was a wise decision.

There are several reasons for the operation to be necessary with symptoms which can vary considerably. There can be severe constipation over several days necessitating strong measures to relieve the condition. There can be constant diarrhoea when the patient may cut down on food in the hope that this will remedy the problem. There can be signs of blood being passed, which is often ignored if the patient has haemorrhoids which may bleed occasionally, especially if he is very constipated. There may also be a constant feeling of nausea and excessive gaseous eructations. All these symptoms should be referred to the GP for him to investigate thoroughly. If he feels that further investigation should be necessary, then an appointment is made with a Consultant at the nearest hospital.

Usually the first consultation is made through an outpatients department and ideally the Stoma Care Nurse would like to meet the patient when the consultant sees him pre-operatively. This will help the patient to settle down to ward routine if he has to enter hospital, for the Stoma Care Nurse will be someone he has met before entry.

The Stoma Care Nurse will have received notification of new entries and will be able to arrange pre-operative visits to the Ward. If the patient has any problems at this juncture, he is able to put them to the Ward Sister or the S.C.N., who will be able to advise or put them in touch with the right helpers. Most of these services are dealt with in other chapters of the book. The list of new patients for the S.C.N. to see would include anyone who has already had a stoma operation, although they may be in for another reason.

In this way the S.C.N. is in touch with all the stoma patients in the hospital. She will guide the patient through all the early stages discussing if the patient so wishes the type of appliance and general management, although sometimes this is left until later. She will visit the patient daily after the operation up to the time they leave hospital to return home.

If, however, the patient has been admitted suddenly as an inpatient, the Ward Sister, who will be in direct charge of the patient under the Surgeon, and her staff are quite used to dealing with any problems which may arise. The expertise of the Ward Sister is of paramount importance for she will have dealt with many stoma cases and will be able to reassure the patient about the medical side of the operation. There is a well-worked out caring system for the new ostomist in which relatives are able to discuss freely with the surgeon, Ward Sister and the S.C.N. all the future implications of an individual case. Further information about the Ward Sister and the S.C.N. will be found on pages 53 and 54 of the book.

Common Questions

When I started to visit patients in their homes I was amazed at the number of wives, husbands, relatives — together with those involved with the patient professionally — who asked question after question. Much of the information required was primarily about nutrition, after which came questions about the disposal of bags, skin problems, obtaining replacement prescriptions for appliances, and about aids to control bowel motion (which many patients did not even know existed).

Marital problems, personal relationships and simply loving another person came to the fore when it was realized that I, too, was a quite normal being with normal emotions.

Many of my fellow colostomists who had had ideas of producing a factual record of help and hints, somehow never had the time in their own renewed busy life. Some of these colostomists returned to office, factory and shop life, some were pilots, sailing instructors, ballet dancers, teachers, executives, engineers, physiotherapists, doctors, dentists and many other demanding occupations, like being a housewife with children to care for, guests to entertain, and — most important — a spouse to love.

So, as my own busy life is easing somewhat, I feel that this record must be made now, for the number of people needing simple advice is increasing all the time. If I can go some way to filling the gap between the very good medical advice available and the need to cope with the day-to-day problems involved in living with a colostomy, then this contribution will be more than worthwhile.

The Major Problem

Everyone must acknowledge the fact that the unnatural way of disposing of the body's waste matter constitutes a problem, in one way or another. The main object is to reduce that problem to the minimum, until one no longer feels that having an opening in the abdomen is antisocial.

In fact, this predominant fear gradually disappears. At first there will be a few hours each day when one is not aware of being different, and as time goes by many do not even remember that they have a stoma, once the main actions of the day have been performed. After all, everyone has to get rid of body waste, and many without a colostomy have their problems, too.

Make no mistake, however, it is up to the patient himself to reach this state, all other medical conditions being equal. Hygiene, nutrition, appliance and skin care have all to be considered. There is not any one appliance or method which is suitable for everybody, any more than there is one diet which is perfect for everyone.

The prime factor to remember is to keep everything as simple and as near natural as possible, for this will eventually give the independence for which everyone strives. The more the patient is dependent on drugs, creams, appliances and aids as a necessity to everyday life, the more he is reminded of the operation.

A Realistic Approach

In talking to those who have had the operation, the first desire is for it to be ignored and for everything to be as before; to have as little change as possible in their way of life. Yet, the patient must grasp the fact that there will be changes, just as there have been physical changes through the operation.

Once this idea has registered with the patient, it is of paramount importance that all those who have not had the operation, but who are endeavouring to help, should remember to impress upon the patient that there are certain things which can be done and certain things which definitely cannot be done.

Firstly, what goes **in** must, in part, come **out**, and you do not have to have had a colostomy to know this. Some people are surprised to think that what they eat and drink can make any difference to their output, therefore much importance should be given to **what** and **how** a patient eats. This need not be a chore, for most people would rather have an untroubled motion than to eat what they like and have problems later.

The question of food is dealt with in the next chapter, for vintage colostomists know that diet comes before appliances. Your appliance or method of management depends upon your normal motion, rather than the other way round.

Secondly, two points which worry patients are odour and flatus (gas). Unless other medical considerations are involved, these two conditions can be dealt with usually by diet and non-drug 'bulkers'. There are two kinds of odour; odour from the waste matter, and odour from flatus. However, these problems will be dealt with in Chapter 1 on nutrition.

After the patient has returned home and some of the functional difficulties have been tackled, there is the underlying worry all the time, especially after the convalescent period has passed, of what their physical and sexual life is likely to be. This is an area in which it is most difficult to help, but — on the other hand, it is most important. This is a problem which tends to emerge after the patient has been home for some time, all the more so if he or she has no one to discuss the matter with. Some problems of this kind are discussed in Chapter 4, and some useful addresses are listed towards the end of the book.

Help and Advice
It should be remembered that each patient is an individual with his or her own particular problems and with different degrees of tolerance to the operation.

The most important aspect to understand is that in all situations the spouse, relative or adviser must show patience, particularly in the early days, tolerance for those who cannot accept the operation, and endless help to those who cannot find the right answer immediately. There must also be patience on the part of the colostomist, for there are more things to contend with than simply disposing of a bag and replacing it.

Once a patient has left hospital, and is without the constant professional care of surgeons, stoma-care nurses, and ward sisters and nurses, the real shock of the operation strikes, and it is often three months or so before the patient can really take in the situation and the advice given in hospital, although medically and surgically he or she has been cleared. This does not mean that the advice is not good — it means, simply, that the patient is still not well enough to absorb the information. This is why, when the patient is in hospital with a colostomy operation as a possibility, the early advice on after-management must be general and thoughtfully given. It has been found, on speaking to many well-recovered colostomists, that it is mainly not until three months after the operation that they are able to take in advice and apply it to their own lives, remembering that each and everyone is different in individual life, age, sexual expectations, and other physical considerations. All these factors must be assessed by those endeavouring to help to rehabilitate the patient to a natural and unfettered life.

The First Few Days at Home

The first two or three days at home are very special. If it is possible, it is a good idea to have a cupboard in the bathroom where all the necessary personal items are kept. I have found that most patients like to have a private place where the 'tools' of their new life may be stored. If this can be done before the patient returns home, then the bags, pouches, creams, and cleaning-up items do not take over the bathroom and intrude upon other members of the family. Any reserves of bags and aids can always be stored in a bedroom drawer, again not letting the bags take over. I have found boxes of bags kept under the marital bed and while this may get them out of sight, the location does not necessarily get them out of the spouse's mind!

Patients who are married could be reasonably expected to have a week or two at home in convalescence, during which time they can begin to find their way in looking after themselves — learning about the disposal of appliances, trying out the diet, and, of course, resting in their own room if this is possible.

Home Help

On returning home it is more than likely that the patient will not feel like doing very much about the house and now would be the time to call upon the Home Help Service, through the local Social Services Department if the family cannot manage. This help can be asked for while the patient is in hospital through the medical social worker, or the stoma-care nurse. The tasks undertaken by the hard-working band of home-helpers have to be experienced to be fully appreciated.

This service provides practical caring support for those of any age who, through illness, age or handicap, find it difficult to look after themselves or their homes.

The criteria on which the amount of help is arranged and the possible costs, vary throughout the country. Those seeking assistance are therefore again advised to contact their local Social Services Department once they return home from hospital, to make quite sure that the authorities understand their need.

Not only are patients encouraged by the knowledge that their homes are maintained to their own standards, but also by the presence of the home-helps, who are sensible, adaptable and caring people. Patients may find it useful to know that they can also apply for aid for their dependants whom they are unable to support while they are convalescent, for this can be an added anxiety to the new colostomist.

Meeting People Again

Very often the most simple activities seem a major effort, meeting friends in one's own home for the first time after the operation, possibly friends who do not fully understand the colostomist's new way of life, and perhaps the patient is fearful of them detecting odour or of having a sudden and unpredictable noisy escape of flatus. This is one of the first steps in rehabilitation — having to meet one's old acquaintances. After this first encounter, a little confidence is installed, followed by a visit to the shops. The people you meet outside may have missed your not being around, but they may not know the cause. Just carry on as before; do your necessary shopping, then visit shops for a look round. Do not feel that people will avoid you because of the operation. This is a very mistaken idea and can cause much anxiety.

Visits to the hairdresser, with the need to bend over a basin for your hair to be washed, can be an even more daunting prospect, but once you have gained confidence this will no longer present a problem to you. Make no excuses for odour or noisy wind. Either ignore it or joke about it.

Making Journeys

Some colostomists hesitate before going on a bus. It is a real step in the early days to travel in public, for most of us fear that if there is a gassy odour the person sitting near us will be conscious of it. The noisy flatus is not, of course, so obvious in these circumstances, but if the colostomist can sit with the stoma away from the other passenger, then any embarrassing incident may be minimized. Also by sitting upright in a comfortable position, flatus is not forced out of the stoma.

When travelling any distance by bus or train, it is always prudent to take a couple of spare bags, or dressings with tissues for cleaning the stoma. The tissues can be disposed of by flushing away in the lavatory. Ladies can always use sanitary bags provided in some toilets, or keep a small brown paper bag or small plastic bag for such an emergency. The appliance may then be folded, wrapped up and placed in the sanitary bin provided.

Men do not always have a bin available in lavatories, but if the used bag or dressing is folded and wrapped up and sealed, it may be left in the corner of the closet or placed in an outside litter bin. There have been efforts to have bins placed in men's lavatories, but without success. However, there is no need to walk around with a soiled bag in a pocket or handbag. Most councils approve of the dressings being placed in a dustbin or litter bin, if the soiled item is folded and well wrapped.

Keys for Public Toilets
See page 82.

Medical Supplies
All patients leaving hospital should have a supply of pouches and aids used in the hospital. This supply should be sufficient to cover the period during which a prescription for everything needed is being ordered from the local chemist. All patients are entitled to have free prescriptions and the form for exemption from prescription charges may be obtained from a General Post Office. The patient does not have to go into details with the counter clerk: just ask for a Prescription Charge Exemption Form.

While a patient is in hospital everything is done for him, and full details of the medicines and appliances should be obtained before leaving. It is important that it is understood how to use the medicines properly, especially the non-drug aids which create bulk and help to firm the motion. If care is not taken with 'bulkers' the reverse effect can occur.

After the Operation
Most patients do not wish to return from the hospital and disappear into limbo, the land in which some hope to hide from everyone the fact that they have an artificial anus and an unusual way of disposing of the waste of the body. I have known patients who feel that they are revolting to themselves and therefore must be revolting to everyone. Many of these patients may have no odour problem, but the very function of disposal is to them unsocial, and they imagine that this makes them socially unacceptable to others. I cannot stress too much that once

the initial effort is made by the patient to go out into company and meet other people, then life can become normal and fulfilling.

Most people when they have had a spell in hospital come home in a mild state of shock, but when one has had any major operation, this condition may persist for a while. This is a difficult period of adjustment for the colostomist and it is during this time that much patient, loving care is needed. Much of the advice given in the early days has not been absorbed, and only begins to make sense when the patient is home and having to work out for himself the best way of dealing with the stoma.

It must also be remembered that everyone may have stomach upsets, either through a virus, wrong food or emotional problems at some time or another, so it is very important for the colostomist to realize that while he is sorting out the foods which are right for him, he may be in touch with people who have a virus, and the motion may be loose for no apparent reason. It happens to the best of us, and it is usually nothing to worry about as the condition will not persist.

When the patient is in hospital a transparent adhesive bag, either closed or open-ended, is placed over the stoma so that the surgeon and staff can see the condition of the stoma, and to have warning when the action may start. This may take a few days after the operation, for the body has to make many adjustments before it can accept food and once again perform to produce waste matter. After food has been consumed and the intestine starts to work again, there may be a change in the type of appliance suggested by the stoma-care nurse or staff in consultation with the surgeon. In the early days in hospital the motion may be loose, somewhat pale and irregular. This output will improve as days go by when the diet is gradually varied, and the patient's general condition improves.

Community Services

From the time the patient returns home the general practitioner and the community nurse will be the caring people with whom easy contact may be made between the regular check-up visits to the surgeon. The community-aid organization is nation-wide and can provide many kinds of help in an emergency.

The doctor and the community nurse should have received notice of the return home of the patient, apart from a letter which is usually given to the colostomist to hand to his or her doctor when they get back. In some areas it is possible for arrangements to be made for the stoma-care nurse to make a domicilary visit through the Community Service.

Also some Community Services provide a free and voluntary laundry service in the event of an emergency. Laundry is collected from the patient's home, taken to the hospital laundry, laundered and returned to the patient. The community nurses do a wonderful job and are especially helpful if the patient is elderly and living in an isolated village or small town. The Community Nursing Officer in the area should also be approached regarding the procedure to obtain help from such organizations as Cancer Relief or Marie Curie.

Just as there may be occasions when the voluntary laundry service may be urgently needed, so it is possible, through the community nurse, to arrange for the local Council to collect dressings, bags and other soiled items. These are placed in a specially supplied plastic sack and collected by the Council, but it must be remembered that this is not the usual way of disposal, only in the case of illness or an emergency.

Progressing with Confidence
Once again, remember that emotional and nervous anxiety can retard improvement. Always look forward and have confidence that you will be able to cope.

As days go by, the medical staff will feel that the patient may return home or leave the hospital confines for a convalescent home. By this time the motion will begin to settle down with a fairly predictable time of action during twenty-four hours, but if the patient nibbles between proper mealtimes and does not consider the type of food and drink consumed, then there may be more than two or three motions a day and the looser the motion, the more frequent it will be. However, a pattern of daily times for the main motion does emerge, whatever may happen in between times, and when this has been established, one can then have confidence in being more adventurous in activites; diet and the type of appliance. This settling down period may take a little time, possibly three to six months, depending upon the patient's attitude to the operation, so be confident that things do improve.

Firm, Not Constipated

Many patients worry that they may become constipated. The possibility of this, in ordinary circumstances, is far less likely than the patient having a loose motion. (By 'too loose' I mean a toothpaste consistency.) The motion must be firm, and the firmer the faeces, the less odour and mess there will be to clean from the skin and bag. A firm motion will avoid skin problems, odour and much worry about the disposal of the bag or dressing. This is one of the points which is not understood: having a firm motion does not mean being constipated.

All waste matter from the body is transmitted by a muscular action through the intestine to the rectum. Before the removal of the rectum, muscles indicated to the patient that a motion would take place. However, with the removal of the rectum and this muscle, the alarm trigger does not work in the same way, and unless the motion is firm, will give little or no indication that a motion is being passed into the bag or dressing. However, with firm faeces there is a sensation which does indicate that something is happening, and as time goes by, the well-recovered colostomist learns to read the signals.

Achieving firm faeces is the one safe way to obtain control of the colostomy, so that the patient controls the output, not the colostomy controlling the patient. If the motion is firm up to a walnut-sized shape, then it is about right. The colostomist is only constipated when the waste matter is obviously waiting to be discharged and he cannot achieve this function. This discharge can soon be encouraged by extra water, vegetables and fruit juice, but it must be remembered that there are many feet of intestine for the food to travel through before the waste is eventually excreted, so do not expect a constipated condition to be remedied immediately, as indeed it could not be if one were constipated without a colostomy.

It is understandable that colostomists fear having a blockage, for this may have been the condition with which they entered hospital, but it is the lack of understanding that a firm action is not constipation, which prevents many patients from reaching the ultimate control in their new way of life. This is a fact which is not appreciated by the new colostomist, for it is very seldom mentioned to a patient unless he talks to a fellow colostomist, who knows only too well that the borderline is very fine between being able to control the output and letting it control them.

Very often, only one very small, unexpected change in habit, diet or emotional trauma can cause a change in the whole body's function resulting in a change in the motion. One does not have to have a colostomy for this to happen, but the colostomist is usually far more aware when this is going to happen and can take evasive steps. When the motion begins to be smelly and gassy, and the consistency softens, then it may take a few hours to get back to 'normal', but a little upset is nothing to worry about.

An old friend of mine, a well-known market gardener who produced exotic plants, said when I asked him how to keep some of his beautiful specimens, 'If the soil is too wet, you'll kill it. If it is just moist, leave it, it's just right. If the soil is too dry, water it, and only then.' I have thought about this old country wisdom and realized how helpful this advice could be to the colostomist. If the motion is too loose, firm it. If it is just moist but firm, it is about right. If it is very dry, then take water, fruit juice, or any other food which is known to be loosening. The amount needed will be a very individual thing.

Minor Problems

There are of course some colostomists who for various reasons cannot reach a state where a motion is firm and there are many ways in which these patients can be helped, especially in the early days after returning home. This is where the right type of appliance and advice can give confidence.

It may take several months before the correct balance of a full life can be obtained, and the many times when despair seizes hold of one must be regarded as a temporary condition and, although I know this may seem easy to say, the present so often seems to be the final state but nothing lasts forever and desperate situations do pass.

I would like to give one instance where the colostomist has the advantage over the non-colostomist! Since my operation some twenty-three years ago, I have had very good health, but I have had during that time three attacks of influenza, with the attendant problems of the disease. Of course, during the illness one does not want to eat, yet vast quantities of bags are used every day, but while other members of the family and friends are laid low for some three weeks, the colostomist gets over this type of tummy problem much more quickly. In fact, I anticipate being out of normal work for about three or four days only. This is a fact borne out by many vintage colostomists, who do not have other medical problems apart from the colostomy.

Many new patients find it difficult to accept the fact that even an 'old' colostomist can have tummy upsets — they imagine that once the motion is firm and able to be dealt with, then there will not be problems at any time thereafter. This is not realistic. Everyone, colostomist or otherwise, can have flu or a stomach upset through no fault of their own, and when this happens, colostomists must accept the fact and take the right steps to help themselves and, if they need help, to ask for it from the GP, consultant or stoma-care nurse at the hospital.

Phantom Pains

Another problem, often early in convalescence, is the feeling of phantom pain in the rectal area, where the rectum has been removed. One has often heard of a patient who has had a leg removed complaining of pain in a non-existent calf or foot; these are called phantom pains because they appear to have their source in a part of the body that has been removed.

Similar sensations can occur with the removal of the rectum. It can happen early on in convalescence or later on when other muscles in the lower part of the body become slack, and this can happen if insufficient exercise is taken. Even the person who is arthritic and cannot move much should endeavour to move about a little and keep all the working parts of the body going.

The activation of phantom pains can occur even quite late in the life of a colostomist; it can be caused through an energetic sneeze, or simply over-eating when used to a small food intake. A distended stomach, whatever the cause, can cause pressure on the lower muscles which are doing overtime anyway since the removal of the rectum and supporting muscles.

It is important for the patient to know that this can happen, even after some years, for if it happens unexpectedly much mental anxiety can be caused. This feeling is very real and the colostomist may well wonder if the pain, rough sensations and bearing-down feeling, means that all is not well and the prime cause for the operation has recurred. Simple phantom pains are common, so do not feel over-concerned, but if they persist, ask for the reassurance of your GP or surgeon.

However, it has been found that if, at the beginning of the sensations, a woman can use a vaginal whirl spray with water as cool as may be acceptable to the vagina, to be used over a period of two or three days, using the spray at least night and morning, it will reduce the pain, which gradually will disappear. Those colostomists who have tried this hydrotherapy have found it very beneficial. For the man who can also get these pains, it is very helpful for the whole of the rectal area to be sprayed with cool water, at least twice a day until the sensation disappears. Do not use hot water, for this will not bring about the desired result. A simple bath-spray of the type which is fixed to the taps for hair-washing, is quite suitable, so long as the spray is directed to the right part of the anatomy.

It is not known why this helps, but it can be attributed to the activation of the muscles in the lower part of the body so that they can once again work correctly, reducing the pressure upon the lower spine and remaining muscles.

Sometimes a man can get these sensations when he has a slight urine imbalance and while this very normal problem is being dealt with by the GP, he can use the shower or spray therapy to tone up the muscles.

Baths and Showers
In hospital the patient will have had baths and been told that there is no reason why he should not bath every day. Many patients do not realize when they reach home that they can take a bath without wearing an appliance. The water will not enter the stoma — this cannot happen. Once one has settled down to a regular time of evacuation a bath can be taken quite safely without a bag or dressing, and if one feels uncertain about a possible motion, it is a good idea to keep a packet of paper tissues or a roll of toilet

paper by the bath to meet such an emergency. (Do not use the strong, men's tissues as they do not disintegrate in the lavatory pan easily — after all, they are supposed to be water-resistant as handkerchiefs, and they can cause blockages in the plumbing system.) So, enjoy a relaxing bath, and feel the freedom of being without an appliance for a while.

A bath is very beneficial to the whole tone of the body. If a patient is unable to sit in a bath, a shower is very helpful. This is the only way some patients can feel the benefit of water upon the body, and it is well worthwhile for a shower to be arranged for those who cannot take a full bath. There are many types of caravan showers which can be adapted to the immobile patient; these showers require very little plumbing and are fairly inexpensive.

Support Girdles and Tights

As the patient gets older, the muscles become slacker, and often the tummy drops a little. This can give a full feeling above the stoma. When this happens, the colostomist who has not been wearing any kind of girdle or pantee-girdle should try to find a firm support. Lycra is a good soft material which is firm without being restrictive, and is suitable for both men and women. If a patient has to wear a full appliance all day, then a lycra belt can be adapted by making a hole for the bag. If a small pouch, dressing or stoma cap is worn during the day, after the main evacuation, there is no need to cut a hole. The girdle will keep the stomach in and help to train the tired muscles to hold the waste matter in the new storage space in the colon. Some patients feel cautious about wearing a pull-on belt, and long after it is really necessary, still wear a surgical belt. Of course some patients for other reasons have to wear this type of support, but many colostomists do not need anything more than a light girdle, and this gentle support will not cause any harm to the stoma and its proper function.

Another good idea for holding a dressing, small bag or stoma cap in place, and to give a sense of security and support, is to wear a pair of support tights. The gusset can be removed if necessary, and I know some men who have adapted their wives' laddered tights for their own use. A well-known chemist, with branches in most towns, produces a good and reliable line in support tights, with a really well supported pantee section, made up to quite a large hip size. This is particularly helpful to men for they have to wear trousers, supported by a belt or braces, underpants and, under that, the appliance with a belt and a possible skin aid, so anything which cuts down the bulk and pressure on the stomach must be seriously considered. There are other suggestions in the chapter on appliances, but this is very much a personal and individual preference. I heard the other day that cricketers and athletes in training use support tights, and they are not embarrassed about it: so gentlemen-colostomists would be in good company.

The pantee-girdles made by another well-known firm with branches in most towns are very suitable for they are made up to quite a large size. When purchasing girdles or tights, it is wise to get one size larger than previously taken. If they prove too large, they can easily be exchanged.

Some support tights have a heavy seam which can cause irritation and soreness of skin between the thighs and in the rectal area. By turning the tights inside out the seam does not come in contact with the skin, and very often the texture of the tights is softer if worn this way.

It is also quite a good idea to turn pantee-girdles inside out as the seams can cause irritation, especially if the patient has to sit for long periods.

Sometimes, after the operation, the waist line is increased, especially if the stoma is high in the abdomen. This can make the comfortable fitting of a skirt-band difficult. It is suggested that by using velcro the waist size can be varied according to the appliance worn, food consumed and the type of underwear, which can change with the seasons.

Backache

After the operation many patients find they have a constant backache and while other problems push this into the background for the time being, it is a condition which should be investigated fairly soon, for usually backache does not go away. The very nature of the operation and the way in which it has to be performed does put the back under strain, especially if there has been a previous history of back problems.

Sometimes this is put down to rheumatism, but it has been found that if a patient has to sit around during convalescence, the back condition is aggravated, remembering of course that the bottom is probably sore anyway for some weeks. When the patient feels able to seek advice about this, he should do so as soon as possible, either from the GP, surgeon, or the hospital, or through private practice and techniques, such as an officially registered chiropractor or osteopath.

Those who have backache and a colostomy or ileostomy should have no fears about having treatment from a fully qualified and registered manipulative consultant, for he will have had experience in helping those with a stoma. (I have had back treatment when necessary for the past fifteen years.)

One other simple and very important hint is for the patient to sit properly, for this will help both the backache and the adjustment of the body to the stoma. Everyone should sit in a comfortable upright chair, with their knees at right angles to the body with the feet firmly placed upon the ground. In this way the body is correctly supported by the spine and this will prevent any strain upon the back and will also prevent the stomach being bent over and twisted or creased, which can cause a quick passage of flatus. If the patient wishes to sit in an easy chair, then place an extra four inches or so of foam cushion on the seat, so that the knees are at right angles to the back and the feet are flat on the ground.

1.

NUTRITION

In the past few years the question of nutrition has been constantly in the news. It is hardly possible to open a newspaper, look at television or listen to radio without the question of food and drink being regularly discussed. This is a subject which many nutritionists and dietitians have been trying to get over to the public for years so this new interest in food and drink could be a great advance in changing attitudes and encouraging healthy eating habits. This is an important step in preventive medicine. The kind of petrol put into one's car is that suitable to the engine, yet in the past little thought has been given to the kind of fuel put into the most precious possession we have — Ourselves.

In making some 400 visits to ostomists during the year prior to the writing of this book, a survey was made of the questions asked and the kind of problems ostomists had with their food intake. The most experienced ostomists were very helpful in their comments and in the following pages these observations have been noted so that their experiences may be of help to others starting out after the operation.

It is obvious that everyone is different, with or without a stoma. Hippocrates observed some 400 years BC and Lucretius said in

Roman times that, 'one man's meat is another man's poison', so intolerance to some foods is nothing new. I do feel that the following ideas can help ostomists to come to their own decision about the foods they can tolerate and to be aware of some of the common pitfalls.

Some ostomists claim they can eat anything, then go on to say '. . . but of course I avoid foods which are smelly or can cause an upset, or give me an evacuation problem'. Don't we all! This comes down to having a good look at the foods we eat and observing the results and acting upon them, remembering that, of course, the choice is the ostomist's own decision.

There are as many schools of thought about the approach to nutrition as there are to appliances, but it is very often when the patient has been home for a while that he realizes that there is more to management than sticking on a bag and then disposing of it.

Psychologically, it is said to be bad to tell a patient not to eat certain foods because it is thought that it will cause them distress if they have to forgo things they like. In practice it is far worse to have to contend with soiled beds, clothes and offensive odours and gas, and to imagine that this is how it is to be from now on, than to exercise a modicum of discipline over the food intake, so that eventually the action is formed and odourless. The patient who exercises a little discipline has a sense of achievement instead of revulsion for themselves and everything to do with the operation, however good the surgery and the prognosis may have been.

Apart from the obvious unpleasantness of a loose action, there is much more involved, especially for a married colostomist. So, all other medical conditions being taken into consideration, the intake of food must be regarded as being of paramount importance.

Finding the Right Nutritional Balance

The word 'diet' is worth looking at. The accepted definition of the word is 'a way of feeding'. In recent years, however, diet has been associated with restricting the body intake to certain foods to produce a loss in weight. So the use of word 'diet' in the management of a colostomy must be thought about very carefully.

It does not mean restricting foods to reduce weight, but rather a nutritional regime followed to obtain a natural and full intake of acceptable foods to the individual body so that it is nurtured and healthy. This can be achieved by an intelligent and observant approach to all food and an acceptance that there is not any one diet which is right for everyone. Both appliance and food is a matter of trial and possible error, until the right balance is found, but both are interrelated.

There is another school of thought which says that a patient should carry on as before the operation, eat what they like and if it does not suit them, then leave it off the menu. Well, it is not as simple as that, either. Imagine the problems to which this can lead. The patient who has been used to sausages, baked beans and fried onions, or the gourmet who likes rich, spiced foods and wines, and the man who has always had his pints of beer every night, thinks that 'carry on as before' means just that, until the next day or two! Anyone who advises a patient to carry on as before without giving some guidance about what can be consumed safely and the known hazards of certain foods, is doing the surgeon and the patient a great disservice, for if there are accidents and upsets, possibly during the night or when outside, patients feel that it is the disease which intially hospitalized them that is causing the trouble, and that the operation has been a failure. Often they do not realize that it could be food and drink which is the reason. This worry has been mentioned to me so many times and is an immediate and not unreasonable reaction to an early disaster.

So we must come to the conclusion that only well-recovered colostomists, who have experimented with their diet and management, really know the anxieties and hazards to be met. In other words, being on the receiving end is the only way for all colostomists to judge what is right for them and this has to be ascertained after the operation, when the system has settled down to being receptive to food again. Do not accept the 'carry on as before' philosophy, for this is not based on experience or fact. Adjustments have to be made and there is only one person who can do that — the colostomist himself, by applying his experience, and the knowledge of other colostomists. The patient who has had to cope with uninformed advice will take a lot of convincing and encouragement to go forth again to meet the world, however well meant the advice may have been.

Experimenting with Food Combinations

If one food does not seem to agree, then it should be left alone for a while, but any food which has an adverse effect on the motion should not be banned forever. There are so many circumstances when a food may be consumed which can produce an adverse reaction in the bowel, while it may be perfectly acceptable in other conditions. For instance, there may be some combinations of food which are very good and nutritious and completely acceptable to the individual, but if some of these foods are taken in combination with other items or drink, an apparently inexplicable looseness of the motion may be produced.

When returning home from hospital, one often does not feel like preparing a meal during this convalescent period, and it can be difficult for the spouse to produce a meal which would be appetizing. Now would be the time to start from scratch by having a simple meal of meat or fish, which is usually acceptable to most colostomists, with fresh potatoes and possibly carrots, with gravy if desired. Gravy can sometimes be unpredictable, so avoid any which is highly spiced or contains onion. From this simple type of meal, which can be followed with cheese and biscuits, or a sponge pudding for sweet, but avoiding tinned fruit in the first few weeks, the next few days can be experimental, trying out one new vegetable at a time, giving each a couple of days to show some indication of its acceptability. This experimental period is well worth the effort, if effort it may be called, for most of these simple meals consumed in the early days may be taken by the whole family without it appearing to be a special diet for the convalescent patient, who does not usually feel like a fussy meal anyway.

One mistaken idea which many colostomists have is that in the early stages everything consumed must be bland and of a sloppy consistency. This is not so, unless there is another reason for such a diet being prescribed by the doctor. The body needs to have work to do, even though an operation has been performed, and there must be substance or fibre upon which the muscular action can work. So meals of, say, soup, or a mashy stew, followed by rice pudding should be avoided as there is very little fibre content.

Bulkers

While the colostomist will, of course, endeavour to regulate the motion by natural means suitable to themselves, there are aids which will be invaluable at sometime or other. These are known as 'bulkers'. They are non-drugs which form bulk and, particularly in the early days, patients find them very helpful. Methylcellulose in tablet form is one of the most successful means of taking these 'bulkers', for these tablets, although quite large, can be broken up into six or so pieces, and must then be chewed if possible with half a wineglassful of water half an hour before food, after which no liquid should be taken before eating. The tablet must not be swallowed whole, otherwise it will arrive at the other end in the same state! The reason for not taking further drink before eating is that the 'bulker' swells in liquid, and if taken before a meal with as little water as possible, it will absorb moisture during the digestive process and thereby firm the motion. If a large drink is taken with the tablet, or immediately after, then the 'bulker' will absorb this drink and be unable to fulfil its purpose in firming the motion.

The number of tablets taken can vary from one to three before a meal. In the initial stages it has been found that, properly broken up before being taken, about two before each meal of the day is sufficient to regulate the motion in the early days. The tablets can be reduced to one a day, stepping up the intake at the first signs of trouble, always remembering to take them with as little water as possible.

There are granules on the market which perform the same function, but on the whole, the tablet is easier to carry in a pocket or handbag and less inclined to stick to false teeth. The granules also tend to swell too quickly in the mouth and become difficult to swallow. The patient is, therefore, more inclined to swallow extra air with the granules, thereby creating a problem of flatus.

All patients, when they leave hospital and return to their GP, should have a supply of these 'bulkers', for it is better to be prepared for initial and temporary upsets which can be remedied by the use of this simple non-drug. Also the firming of the motion will help to avoid skin problems and assist in a quick recovery.

What Happens When We Eat

I think it would be helpful to consider briefly what happens when we eat and why it is necessary for food to be well chewed at the beginning of its journey. The small intestine, which is the first part of some thirty feet of intestine ending in the rectum, receives food from the stomach by way of a muscular movement called **peristaltic action**. This movement must be kept healthy by giving it work to do, for as with any other muscular system, if it is not used properly it will fall into a passive state. This is why fibre is so necessary in the diet, for if the muscular system does not have something to work on, then the digested food will pass through in a semi-formed state, causing problems at the end of its journey.

The end of the small intestine is called the ileum. This is very important in the absorption of food into the body, and it is from this point that the remainder of the food will pass on into the large intestine which is about the last nine feet of the whole intestine. This length of intestine, which is also known as the colon, surrounds the small intestine and it is this last section which absorbs the liquid from the bulk passing through. Because a length of this colon has been removed in a colostomy operation, the faeces passing along will obviously be looser than those in a normal action.

By the regulation of food and by taking in extra fibre to help form a firm motion, the body's muscular action is kept healthy and working in a normal way. If a bulker is taken as described, it is already in the stomach, waiting to absorb the liquid which then forms bulk to help the food through the system, and it does not interfere with the natural absorption of nutrients in the food.

As time goes by and the muscular system starts working efficiently, less ' bulker' is needed and should be taken only when the food is suspect and may cause a problem. One of my own preventive measures is to take a tablet before going out for a meal, either with friends or in an hotel, so that if any unusual or highly spiced food is produced, I do not have to worry about it the next day, and this causes no embarrassment by having to refuse food which may have taken the hostess a long time to prepare. The use of 'bulkers' is very much an individual thing, so they may be experimented with, until the right balance is found, as they are not drugs.

Mastication

All food, especially pulse foods, should be very well chewed. Peas, beans and corn are small and some people are inclined to swallow them whole without chewing, causing much gas and inconsistent motions. The large pulses have to be chewed before swallowing, so they are already broken down for absorption into the digestive system. To avoid undue gas or flatus, food should be put into the mouth and chewed with the mouth shut, and swallowed before placing more food into the mouth. In this way, extra air is not taken into the body at the time of eating. This is very important to remember. Another useful hint in the consumption of food is that one must be sure that not too much of one kind is eaten at any one mouthful. If a meal consists of two or three vegetables with meat or fish, take a little of each on the fork or spoon. Varied foods help the digestive process to deal with the intake. Try not to eat all the root vegetables at one go; mix well, especially when trying out a new food, with meat, potatoes, and high fibre items. This does not mean mashing up food together, but simply taking a little of each food with each mouthful and chewing it well.

Bran

One of the best means of obtaining sufficient fibre in the diet is to take pure unprocessed bran which can be obtained from any good grocery shop or health store. The unprocessed bran is coarse in texture and is not powdery. The very fine bran is more difficult to eat and is often found to be unpalatable, for it is not easily absorbed in liquids such as gravy, fruit juice, fruit salads, stews, soups and milk, but will float on top. The coarse bran absorbs these liquids and those unsuspecting members of the family who say they cannot tolerate bran, will not be conscious of it being introduced into the cooking. It is of great benefit to the whole family, but invaluable to the colostomist.

It is commonly thought that bran must be taken in the morning with cereals or even alone with milk and sugar. This is wrong.

Bran should be taken throughout the day in small quantities, even a teaspoonful with each meal, sprinkled on vegetables or fruit — in fact, on anything. The constant fibre content of the diet, maintained over twenty-four hours, will make the motion as standard as possible.

It is a good idea to put out the daily requirement of two or three tablespoonsful of bran into a small plastic container on the dining table so that one is able to gauge how much is being consumed every day. In this way it can be sprinkled over the food as well as introducing it into the cooking. Bran is not expensive to purchase, for a large bag will last for several months if put into a large glass or plastic air-tight jar.

Do not worry if there is a full feeling in the stomach when first taking bran. Usually, if the bran is spread over the day, this feeling will soon disappear or will not occur at all.

A *teaspoonful* of bran may be used in the following ways without it being noticeable.

— Over muesli or other breakfast cereal, but not alone.
— On fruit, scrambled eggs, omelette, kippers, fish, minced meat, steaks, cutlets. Use as breadcrumbs.
— In all soups, and meat drinks, and gravies.

A *dessertspoonful* of bran may be used on:

— Stewed fruit, tinned fruits and fruit salads, green salads, fresh fruit, and bland sweets with cream.
—Cottage cheese and curd cheese, and yogurt with fruit.

The difference this makes to the firmness of the motion is so helpful that most patients do not mind forming the habit of taking bran, which after the first few weeks is no trouble at all, for there are so many ways in which it can be introduced.

Root and Green Vegetables

Some root vegetables cause odour if, for example, swedes and parsnips are consumed with sprouts or other greens. It is a fairly reasonable guide to eat potatoes and greens with carrots. If other root vegetables are included in the meal, then do not have greens on that particular day. This is no hardship compared with the problems which could ensue. If you find that you are one of the lucky people who can eat all these foods at one meal without odour, flatus or a loose motion, then of course enjoy them.

Individuals must judge for themselves whether they can eat greens of any type. If they cannot eat greens without an odour from the motion or flatus, which can vary in smell and noise with individuals, then they have to decide for themselves whether they will avoid cooked greens and make up for the nutritional loss in other ways, which is quite easy. Alternatively, eat greens at a time when the loosened output and odour does not matter socially. It is possible to gauge the response to certain foods by taking limited quantities of a new food, introducing this to the established and acceptable items in the diet, and watching the motion over some twenty-four hours.

Onions

There are certain foods which (it has been proved) are hazards and must be approached with caution. Quite often these are foods which in the past were consumed frequently, such as onions. These should not now be consumed whole — one or two at Christmastide or with the occasional ploughman's lunch, perhaps, but certainly not every day. It is the flesh which produces a loose and odorous motion, and much flatus. The whole onion can be put in a stew, producing the flavour, but the flesh should be given to someone else!

Pulses

Pulse foods should also be approached carefully. Baked beans should be eaten in limited amounts and not more than once a week; broad beans should be limited, but not to the same extent as baked beans. Butter beans likewise — these could be alternated with broad beans. Corn on the cob may be consumed once a week or so, but the tinned corn can cause problems to some.

Peas can cause flatus and noise, but not so much odour. I would like to tell of my first introduction to peas and a stoma. I was in hospital awaiting the operation about which I knew nothing, and feeling somewhat bewildered. I was approached from across the ward by a very charming lady who said she had a colostomy some six months previously and was in for a further part of her operation. I asked her about the 'opening'. 'Would you like to see mine!', she said. Somewhat taken aback at this invitation I said with some hesitation, 'Well, yes, thank you very much'. Whereupon we walked over to her bed and she showed me the 'opening' which was covered with a transparent bag. As I gazed at this new sight there was an almighty explosion and the stoma produced one perfectly rounded garden pea, as pure in shape and colour as from the pod! Needless to say, we thought it hilarious and a friendship of some nineteen years was cemented, but my relationship with peas has not been so humorous or lasting.

This incident made me realize very early that food was important, as is the way in which it is consumed. Also another lesson was that there is no room for embarrassment with a colostomy!

Vegetable and Meat Stock

If vegetables cannot be taken without problems, save all the water in which the green vegetables or fruit have been cooked for the family, and use this as stock for soups, pot-roasts (which is a method of cooking a joint in a small amount of water instead of fat), cutlets, steaks and gammon, and of course all variations of stews and the occasional mild curry. Also, save all the water from potatoes, swedes, carrots. In fact, all the root vegetables should be used in this way, for in many cases it is the flesh of a certain vegetable, not the liquid, which can cause odour or a loose motion.

Well liquidized or mashed vegetables emulsified with water will make a wonderful soup; even if certain items cannot be taken whole, there will be less odour and flatus if consumed this way, with of course the sprinkling of bran to give fibre.

In this way it is possible to obtain all the benefit of a normal diet without the possible dramatic after-effects.

Cooking for One

If there is only one person to cook for, it is a good idea to cook the greens, potatoes or other root vegetables for one meal, and to keep the water in a cool place or in the refrigerator. Use the liquid the following day for a stew, soup or casserole with potatoes.

In this way, all the vitamins and nutrients which are in the water and usually strained away at the time of cooking, are conserved and it helps the colostomists to have their full food value, even if they do not have whole root or green vegetables every day.

Further Tips

Having varied food and varied methods of cooking also helps one to obtain an acceptable consistency of output. Too much of the same food for weeks at a time should be avoided. If, come summer, you have a beautiful garden and are drooling for raspberries, strawberries and loganberries with cream, and you are longing to have a feed, do so by all means.

It has been found helpful to take a dry biscuit or cream cracker with the fruit as well as bran, but it would be very unwise to have these fruits every day during the whole season. White sugar with fruit can cause extra flatus; brown sugar is better, as less is needed, and honey is better still. If bread is consumed with fresh fruit, gas and odour can follow. Try the biscuit instead.

If one is staying in a hotel or guest house, it is usually easy to ask for a dry biscuit or just produce your own little bran container and sprinkle it on any suspect goodie which you cannot resist. One important thing to remember if one has consumed a loosening food, is to follow this for a day or two with food which is more binding and while this may mean that the motion for the next day or two will be uneven in consistency, it will help to get back to normal sooner than taking drugs and being worried about the outcome.

It is interesting to note that the muscular action of the intestinal system is activated by a meal. Very often within half an hour of a full meal there could be a motion. This is not the food just consumed but the waste matter already in the lower end of the colon which is being urged forward by the increased muscular action. An important point to keep in mind when tempted to nibble between meals! It could be the answer to many colostomists who say they have five or six little motions a day; many of them are nibblers. Three good meals a day are better than six little ones.

Some colostomists who are at work during the day may not find it convenient to eat a main midday meal, and prefer to have it in the evening with the family. That is fine, but the timing of the motion will be different from that of those who eat a main meal midday. This is just a matter of adjustment.

Timing of Passage of Food

One of the frequent problems I have come across is the colostomist who thinks that cutting out a meal or not eating at all for a day will help the bowel output. This is not so and will cause more odour, flatus and stomach cramp than necessary. If regular meals, even if small (but of the right balance), are consumed, a body rhythm is encouraged and will eventually lead to the patient being able to anticipate when the motion will take place.

The timing of the passage of food through the body will depend upon several things:

1. *The position of the stoma.* If it is on the low left-hand side, then the period of time for food to pass through the body's process will be longer and nearer to that of the non-colostomist. The nearer the stoma is to the high right hand side of the body, the looser and more frequent the output will be. This is simply because the length of intestine through which the food has to pass gets shorter the nearer the stoma is to the right-hand side of the body.

Those who have a low left-hand stoma will probably have had the rectum removed but many feet of intestine left, through which the waste can proceed with the aid of the peristaltic action. These are the colostomists who can obtain a greater control over the motion. It is well worthwhile making the effort to gain this control, for not only does control mean that the odour disappears, but cleaning-up is negligible and the disposal of dressings and bags easier. As a bonus, the smelly flatus can be identified, enabling the offending food to be reduced or omitted from the diet.

The time it takes for odorous gas to be produced can vary with individuals but, generally, colostomists find that the odour ties up with food consumed the previous day. If the motion is of toothpaste consistency the gas usually takes little time and is odorous; and if the motion is firm it usually takes slightly longer to be produced and is not odorous.

2. *Other medical conditions* must be taken into consideration.

3. Too bland foods without fibre (see page 32).

4. Not sufficient food being taken to produce a regular motion. I have visited patients who exist on cream crackers and coffee, or a milky drink, and they wonder why they do not have a regular and firm motion. I was asked by one consultant to see a colostomist who seemed to be worried because she did not have a motion for three days. The answer was that she was not eating enough because she did not want to change her appliance. What she did eat was unbalanced and limited, which meant that the food consumed took longer to produce any waste. This patient was 'booted and spurred' with bags and equipment, which the community nurse came in daily to change, but very often the bag was not even soiled.

This patient thought she was constipated and had not told either the consultant or community nurse that she was not eating. How could she be constipated — there was nothing to be constipated on!

Colostomists should not be frightened of eating anything which is not soft, for some feel that anything which is solid will cause an obstruction, the possible cause of going into hospital in the first place. They may also feel that solid food may cause damage to the stoma, which means that they really do not understand what has happened to their body or how it functions. I repeat this point, at risk of being tedious to some, because it is vital that the simple functioning of the colostomy is understood by the colostomist.

Liquids
There are certain indisputable rules to follow, so let us look at some.

Keeping a Firm Motion
In the early days no liquid should be taken for half an hour before food, especially if any of the known bulkers used to firm the waste output have already been taken half an hour before a meal, for the more liquid taken at this time, the looser the output will be.

On a special occasion a glass or two of wine with food may be consumed, but beer and lager could be a very bad idea for they produce gas and odour, and taken with food can produce a most unfortunate result.

Half an hour or so after food, a cup of coffee or tea may be taken; if away on holiday in a hotel or visiting friends, by the time coffee is served sufficient time may have elapsed to take liquid after the meal. The odd occasion does not matter — it is a constant habit which can upset what could be a normal motion. However, the easy point to remember in the early days is not to take liquid for half an hour before a meal and a similar period after food. After a while this can be adjusted to the individual reaction but, to repeat, no liquid should be taken before food if a bulker has been taken.

Alcoholic drinks should be regarded as a very personal matter. Beer, by virtue of its quantity, should not be consumed daily in large amounts. The odd shandy or pint when a man has to go out with his friends could be acceptable, but if more is consumed, then problems will follow. Two whiskies or gins, with soda water, could be taken without too much reaction, but mineral waters can prove very gassy. 'Slimline' minerals could be the answer for some. Whisky and ginger ale is not a good combination as a regular drink. Some find that red wines cannot be consumed safely without an upset, but generally a medium white wine during a meal causes little loosening of the motion if taken only occasionally.

Brandy as a liqueur, not with a mineral water, is reasonably acceptable, but again is a very personal matter and caution must be observed during the early stages. Sherry within limits does not seem to cause too much trouble.

Many lemonades and fizzy drinks can cause gas and odour. Soda water usually can be taken without trouble, *Perrier* or other natural sparkling waters can be a good standby.

Many drinks like the instant teas, coffees and milks can create a looseness, but it is well worthwhile observing whether this happens, so that other food is not blamed for a problem. Observation can be fascinating and rewarding, for it will eventually mean freedom and a sense of achievement.

Generally, tea, coffee, meaty drinks (*Bovril*) and milky drinks are acceptable.

Obtaining a Loose Motion

This is a very easy matter. If the motion is too firm or does not dispel itself into the bag or dressing without pain or pressure, then an extra amount of water, fruit juice or liquid taken with the methylcellulose tablets, which must be well-chewed or broken-up and swallowed with half a pint at least of liquid (hot tea or coffee), plus an acceleration of green vegetables, will help to get the body action moving. It is much easier to rectify a constipated situation than to ameliorate a loose condition.

Often drugs and medicines taken for another medical condition to which the patient is prone, can cause constipation, and the patient must always remind his doctor that he has a colostomy and that he does not wish to be made any looser or firmer than he is at present. The doctor will then consider this when prescribing medication. I have come across patients who have been prescribed tablets for sciatica and sent to bed for two or three weeks. Some have been constipated for two weeks, producing no motion during that time. Needless to say, there were real problems when the action did start, but if there had been understanding of the colostomy when secondary medication had been given, much misery could have been avoided, including a return to hospital in one of the cases.

In a constipated state, plenty of liquid must be taken, but it will take a little time for the result of liquid or green vegetables to work through the system.

There are of course medicinal aids to prevent constipation, but these are not really the answer, and should be avoided. If the diet is right and the colostomist is reasonably active, there is no reason why constipation should not be rectified by diet and natural methods, if all other medical conditions are taken into consideration.

Dieting to Shed Weight

There are some colostomists who simply have to lose weight and dieting for this purpose is very difficult for a colostomist, for many of the foods which help to gain control of the motion are the fattening ones. I have fallen victim to thinking that cutting out potatoes, bread and living on salads, meat, cheese and fish is something which can be done without a problem, and while this might help those who are not colostomists, it is not necessarily true for those with a stoma, for cutting out many foods without knowing the result can have very unfortunate consequences.

As I have mentioned in the previous section, the muscular action must have something to work on, otherwise the stomach contents just pass straight through. Also, if a weight-losing diet specially designed for the individual is not undertaken, there can be very distressing stomach cramp. To the uninitiated colostomist this may appear to be caused by a more serious condition than the body simply being starved of enough of the right food to keep the intestine active and healthy.

The ordinary diet for slimming is not suitable for the colostomist and needs the individual's very careful observations on the binding and fattening foods which are required but which may be left out of the menu (apart from, of course, sugar, alcohol, sweet foods, chocolate and the known fattening foods which are not necessary, such as cakes, sweet biscuits and butter on cooked vegetables). So every slimming effort for a colostomist must be designed by the colostomist himself.

There are magazines for slimmers, and some produce a wonderfully helpful selection of ideas which can give very exciting menus of nutritious and fibrous meals. By slightly stepping up the calorific value of some of the interesting meals suggested in these magazines, a very normal and healthful regime can be obtained. Many of these meals do not need any special preparation and are very suitable for the individual who is living alone. Where onion is suggested in the recipe, just leave it out or put in the whole onion to give flavour, without eating the flesh. Onion is often suggested in slimming menus because it is loosening and useful in shedding weight. However, extra flavour can be obtained by using herbs and usually herbs are not troublesome.

Bran Tablets
There is a bran-based tablet on the market which is used as a meal substitute. The calorific value is very low and a useful way to use this tablet is to take one or two before the colostomist's slimming meal, thereby replacing some of the fibre which may have been left out, and at the same time keeping the motion firm. This tablet should not be used as a meal-substitute for a colostomist, but

as an aid to take the edge off the appetite, thus making it easier to feel satisfied by a low-calorie main meal.

Rye and Wheat Breads
Some colostomists find that rye and wheat crispbreads cannot provide sufficient fibre when slimming, although in the ordinary slimming menu these crispbreads are a standard food. Bran, bulkers and dry biscuits could substitute for crispbreads, if the brown bread intake has to be cut down, provided that not too much liquid is taken near the meal.

Fruit Juices
Juices without sugar can be taken in moderation, but still observing the rule of no liquid with a bulker before food or sooner than half an hour after. Cutting out a meal during the day in an effort to slim will not help the colostomist. Cut down, but do not cut out, and do play it by ear!

Some Generally Acceptable Foods

Meat

Beef	Liver
Bacon	Lamb
Gammon	Poultry
Ham (not tinned)	Sweetbreads
Kidney	Tripe (no onions — try mushrooms instead)

Usually processed and highly spiced tinned meats must be treated with caution. Pork and pork sausages should not be taken more than once a week. Pork can cause extreme odour. Twice-cooked stews or tinned stew meat contain little fibre and need observation. Paté which contains onion, garlic and spices can cause odour, as can pork pies and steak pies ready-made from the shops.

Fish

All fresh fish	Smoked mackerel
Roes	Smoked salmon
Kippers	Sardines and sprats (do not worry about the little bones — chew well)

Eggs

These may be acceptable to some, but should be tried out by taking two a week. Some people can take one a day without odour. Scrambled or poached eggs usually cause less of a problem, but some eggs should be taken during the week in some form.

Fresh Vegetables

        Potatoes (absorb liquid).

        Carrots.

Limit intake during the week but have some vegetables every day:

Asparagus	Artichokes
Broad Beans	Tomatoes
Courgettes	Turnips
Broccoli	Sprouts
Parsnips	Swedes
Celery	Marrow
Green beans	Mushrooms
Cauliflower	Red and green peppers
Cabbage	Lettuce

Corn on the cob, peas, cucumber should be observed for problems.

Tinned Vegetables

Baked beans	Broad beans
Beetroot	Green beans
Tomatoes	Celery

Caution with these tinned foods.

Milk

This may be taken in all drinks and soups, but do not rely upon milk alone for a meal.

Bread

  Brown bread

  Bran bread or rolls

  Limit crispbreads, white bread and rolls

Butter and Margarines

A polyunsaturate margarine is good. Butter (with white bread) can cause odour and gas, but choice depends very much on individual preference.

Cheese

Brie	Curd
Cheddar	Edam
Caerphilly	Gloucester
Cottage	Leicester

Try making your own mixture with cottage cheese and fruit, but not using onions or nuts. Blue and other similar strains should be tried out with much caution, as some colostomists finds that they cannot tolerate this type of cheese, which results in sore skin around the stoma, quite apart from the disagreeable odour produced. The occasional portion of a blue cheese may be acceptable to some.

Puddings

Milk puddings (if plenty of fibre taken during the meal)
Pastry with brown flour
Sponge puddings
Tinned fruit, after the stoma has settled down
Fresh fruit

Chocolate, rhubarb, plums, gooseberries and any pie filling which is acid or loosening should be included cautiously in the menu, especially if white flour is used.

Prunes and figs are not acceptable.

Sugar

This is a very bad addition to the diet, causing gas and odour. If sweetness is needed in cooking use honey or brown sugar. Sugar should be limited as it causes fermentation in the stomach and the result is odour and flatus.

Salt

Should be limited in all cooking and not sprinkled on food, as apart from it being harmful to the quality of the food, it will create a thirst which means that the colostomist will want to drink more liquid and this will not help the firmness of the waste matter, especially if 'bulkers' are taken, as explained on page 33.

Fresh Green Salads and Vegetables
It is generally thought that pips and skins are bad for the colostomist, but this is not necessarily proved in practice. If lettuce, tomatoes, beetroot and other usual salad ingredients are well cut up and chewed before swallowing, then most patients can eat this kind of meal, remembering to take fibre with the food. Dressings, cole slaw and other made-up salad specialities should be looked at carefully.

Fresh Fruit
Caution should be exercised, but all fruits should be tried over a period of time. Try not to experiment with more than two types a week.

Tinned Fruit
Peaches, pineapple, apricots, fruit salads, with the requisite fibre, are usually acceptable after a period of settling down to the other main items of the colostomist's diet.

Biscuits
Water or cream crackers are good in a limited amount — but not a packet a day! Biscuits with a fat and sweet content are inclined to cause odour and gas if taken in an excessive amount, but three or four a day would be all right.

Cakes
Most cakes should be taken in a cautious way. If white flour and white sugar are used, then gas and odour can follow (not to mention the toppings and fillings), causing a loose motion. However, try out this food, which is not essential but an indulgence, should there be a wild desire to have sweet food. The occasional cake does not matter.

Parsley
Parsley is one of nature's own deodorants. It is easily grown in

a small patch of the garden and will continue for many a year. It can be grown in a large pot indoors, in a sunny window, protected from draughts, and can be purchased all the year round, and will keep in water for two weeks without going yellow. So anyone without a suitable growing area can have the benefit of parsley.

The way this plant is used for a colostomist is as a deodorant, and its qualities are, of course, beneficial to anyone else. It will deodorize offensive tobacco smell, cleanse the breath and deodorize the eventual output.

When I entertain guests for a meal I always have plenty of parsley sprigs on the salad and cheese, so that anyone aware of the benefit of parsley can just take a head or two.

This plant is also a marvellous source of vitamins and may be introduced into many recipes.

Vitamins

Frequently I am asked for a list of foods which produce the essential vitamins and trace minerals so that patients can endeavour to work out a balanced diet for themselves. There are four basic rules to follow in working out a balanced meal.

1. Fruit once a day. Tomatoes may be taken in this category.
2. Root, green or yellow vegetables once a day with a certain amount of salads and raw food, which can be quite acceptable to a colostomist.
3. Meat, poultry, fish, liver, kidneys, eggs or cheese may be taken as desired.
4. Margarine, or butter in small amounts.

Vitamin A: Milk, fish, fish oils, yellow vegetables.

Vitamin D: Fish liver oils, eggs, milk, butter and margarine. Vitamin A and D nearly always occur together in foods.

Vitamin E: Green leafy vegetables; milk, eggs, liver. Vegetable oil margarine, soya bean oil, corn oil, wheat germ oil.

Vitamin K: Green leafy vegetables, pig's liver, alfalfa, eggs and milk contain a small amount. Spinach is also a good source, if it can be tolerated without problems.

Vitamin C: Citrus fruits, tomatoes, parsley, green peppers, green
               vegetables, lettuce, bananas, black berries, apples,
               watercress, mustard and cress, blackcurrants. As
               vitamin C is water soluble, only a small amount of
               water should be used for quick cooking of
               vegetables and fruit, with the lid put on to exclude
               as much air as possible.

Vitamin P: Usually occurs with vitamin C. Paprika is a good
               source.

Vitamin B: Yeast, lean meat, liver, fish roe, kidney, *Marmite*,
Complex: milk, cheese, eggs, wheat germ, leafy vegetables.
               Vitamin B is also water soluble, so only a small
               amount of water should be used in cooking. Save
               all water as stock.

Food Supplements

Many colostomists feel that they need a supplement to their diet,
especially if they have to cut out oranges, apples and certain green
vegetables. The following additions to the daily diet could help.

Vitamin C

Two 50mg tablets taken daily would make up for any deficiency,
and I have also found that since I have taken these easily-obtained
and inexpensive tablets, as I cannot take some fruits, I have not
had colds or catarrh. Many people do not agree that vitamin C
will help with colds, but it works for me and many others.

Kelp (seaweed)

These tablets are a very good source of iodine, which is so
necessary for a healthy diet. Kelp also contains several vitamins
and many other important minerals. If green vegetables are
omitted from the diet, a regular intake of not more than two tablets
a day, with food, will avoid any deficiency. They may be broken
up and swallowed with the meal. There is also a powdered form
to use in cooking (not to be taken instead of tablets) which soon
dissolves in hot food.

Brewer's Yeast

This is a very good source of vitamin B and should also be

regarded as a long-term supplement. Two tablets a day are adequate, if the diet is otherwise reasonably balanced.

If both yeast and kelp are taken daily, it is suggested that they are not taken at the same meal. Some colostomists prefer to take them on alternate days, depending upon their own individual diet, but the important point to remember is to take any food supplement regularly for good results. Vitamin C, kelp and yeast tablets may be purchased inexpensively from the health shops and chemists.

2.

APPLIANCES

At the time I had my operation some twenty-three years ago there were no specially trained nurses in stoma care. The ward Sisters and staff, from their practical experience in caring for colostomy patients as part of their general work, were the most knowledgeable people available, and once a patient was discharged from hospital, the only contact was when making check-up visits to the surgeon, and his staff, whom the patient may or may not have known.

Before leaving hospital, the surgeon had told me that control could be obtained through diet; so armed with this information I returned home to my village. There was a very limited selection of appliances available, the prescriptions took two or three weeks for delivery, and the publicity for new ideas coming on the market was negligible. Because the appliance I was given was neither accident-proof nor comfortable, I soon devised my own type of dressing, based on gamgee and water-proof plaster, which I purchased from the village chemist. By now I had experimented with the diet control idea, and by the time I had returned to hospital for my check-up three months after the operation, I was able to abandon the appliance during the day time. From then on I was requested by the surgeons and nursing staff to see anyone in need of reassurance, both pre- and post-operative, and I still continue to do so.

Post-operative Care and Advice

However, in the meantime, the need for trained staff in stoma care became apparent, and in the past few years stoma-care nurses have been appointed to most operating hospitals. No longer does a patient undergo a colostomy or ileostomy operation without meeting his or her stoma-care nurse, if there is one in the hospital. The Ward Sister may put a patient in touch with a well-recovered colostomist, and the patient is informed of all the help which can be offered. Advice is given on the right choice of appliance, taking into account size, skin condition and any other problem, such as arthritic hands or being partially-sighted, which may make the choice of appliance very important and difficult.

The medical social worker also works in close touch with the stoma-care nurse, and between them they endeavour to make the return home as easy as possible for the new colostomist.

The stoma-care nurses hold clinics to which the colostomist may go for help and advice after they have left hospital, and many nurses can arrange to make domiciliary calls if the patient is unable to get to the clinic.

One very important thing to remember is that a visit from a well-recovered colostomist can prove to be very helpful to the new colostomist, for it is in the early days that problems appear which can be very easily dealt with by advice from someone who has experienced most of these early set-backs. A visit from a fellow colostomist, apart from any advice they may have to offer on the practical side, is very uplifting to the new colostomist for they then realize that it is possible, all other things being equal, to lead a normal life. A visit from a colostomist who is acceptable as a 'visitor' can be arranged by the stoma-care nurse, community nurse or the doctor if this is discussed with him. If a patient, on their return visit for a check-up to the surgeon, wishes to see a colostomist, they should mention this to him so that he can draw on his much wider selection of well-recovered colostomists in whom he has confidence.

There is no need nowadays for anyone to feel that there is no one they can turn to in times of distress.

If a colostomist wishes to know where the nearest Stoma Clinic is to be found, should he move house or live in an isolated district, there is a list which is available free to anyone and is mentioned towards the end of this book under *Useful Addresses,* and is issued by the Royal College of Nursing.

If a patient finds transport difficult, it is a good idea to contact Age Concern or the Red Cross through the local representatives.

Free Prescriptions

Usually the stoma-care nurse informs the community nurse through the patient's doctor or gives the patient a letter to the GP before he leaves hospital, so there should be a continuation of care after leaving hospital. However, it is always advisable to let the doctor know as soon as the patient returns home, for an Exemption Certificate, which has to be obtained for free prescriptions, must be signed by the doctor. It must be remembered that a prescription will soon be needed after the return home for further supplies of appliances and until it is known how long it takes for the local chemist to obtain the goods, one has to be well-prepared with a good supply.

The Exemption Certificate is obtained from a General Post Office (simply ask for it) and does not cause any embarrassment. I have asked for twelve certificates at one time without an eyebrow being raised. Any woman over sixty years or a man over sixty-five does not, of course, pay for prescriptions anyway.

Choosing the Right Appliance

When a colostomist first faces the prospect of a lifetime of having to deal with an unusual way of waste disposal, it is important that he realizes that there is no one appliance suitable for everyone — there are so many different types of stomas, positions of the stoma and primary causes.

Manufacturers are improving appliances all the time. The materials used in the manufacture have advanced so that many bags are now odour-proof and the adhesives are very nearly leak-proof. However, once again, this is an individual approach. Some skins may be perfectly all right, while others are intolerant of the adhesive or plastic material used for the bag. This may be especially so during the hot weather when the body perspires, sometimes stopping the adhesive from adhering to the skin for the usual period. Also, during the hot weather, the plastic may stick to the skin and cause an irritation. One very good tip here is to fold up the bag once, so that the bottom of the bag can be held by a small piece of plaster, thereby keeping half the length of the bag away from the skin. When an action starts, it is always easy to remove the plaster and let the bag down to its full length. Some manufacturers make a washable cover for bags so that the skin is protected; indeed, many patients make their own if they wish to have this protection. Some patients, however, do not wish to have the additional covering because it can look bulky, so using the method described above can overcome this added thickness under clothes.

Many manufacturers have their own nurses in stoma care, and they are only too happy to help if a patient finds the products are not up to standard. In fact, the more information they receive on any problems, the more likely they are to modify their appliances.

There are basically two shapes of bag: the open-ended and the closed bag.

The Open-ended Bag
This is also called a drainable bag and is sometimes used in hospitals to facilitate the emptying of the bag during the early days. This type of bag always has a clip or tie-end and a patient must see that they have a reserve of clips when they return home. I suggest that a small roll of 1-inch waterproof plaster is kept handy so that there is always one way of sealing off the end in an emergency. This is the same plaster which can be used for temporarily reducing the size of the bag, when it is not needed, described above.

Open-ened bags are recognizable by the shape. They are usually longer, either triangular or with an extended open funnel which is folded and clipped (see Figure 1).

These bags are sometimes used by patients who need help with changing a closed bag and, if the action is loose, it can be emptied without removing the bag from the skin. Also, some patients who have a very firm action find it more convenient if they are at work

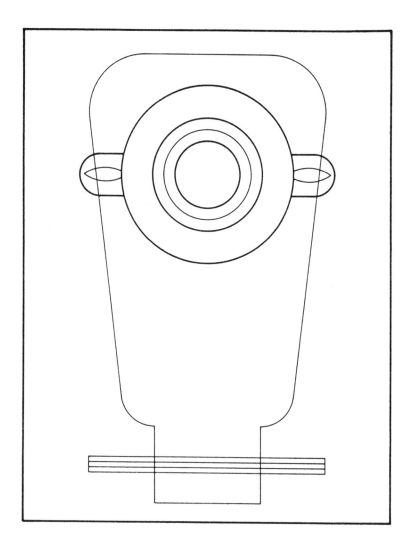

Figure 1. Open-ended with flange to take a belt, and adhesive flange sometimes with a karaya gum ring. Tie or clip must be used to tie the open end.

or unable to make a complete change, to have an open-ended bag. There would be little odour and the firm motion can be easily disposed of in the lavatory in the usual way. This type of bag is also used by ileostomists, whose motion is not so firm as that of a colostomist.

They are produced in odour-proof material and some are attractively patterned, or in an opaque plastic.

The Closed Bag
This is more often used by a colostomist, for as the motion becomes firmer, it is easy to empty the bag. There are many sizes, from a small casual bag which can be used during the day or at any time that the bowel is not likely to work, to a larger one which some patients like to wear during the night, or at work when it may be difficult to change without leaving the factory, office or shop.

Once the motion has settled down, the patient can more or less predict when the main action of the day will take place and can then judge when to use the larger bag or the small pouch.

The smaller pouches are very suitable for those who wish to play sports or swim and as with the open-ended bag, some manufacturers have now produced casual pouches which are opaque or patterned attractively (see Figures 2 and 2a).

Of course, the different manufacturers use a variety of adhesives and this is where the stoma care nurse and experimentation can prove invaluable.

Methods of Colostomy Management
There are, broadly speaking, five known ways of dealing with a colostomy once the patient has been discharged and they are on their own. Most bags described here are produced with an open or closed end. One important point to note at this stage is that all bags are produced in various sizes to suit different stomas, and all bags must a good fit round the stoma (about one-eighth of an inch from the actual stoma) otherwise skin problems can occur, if faeces which are loose touch the stoma and surrounding skin.

Aids to skin and motion control are mentioned at the end of this chapter, but the important thing to remember is to keep all

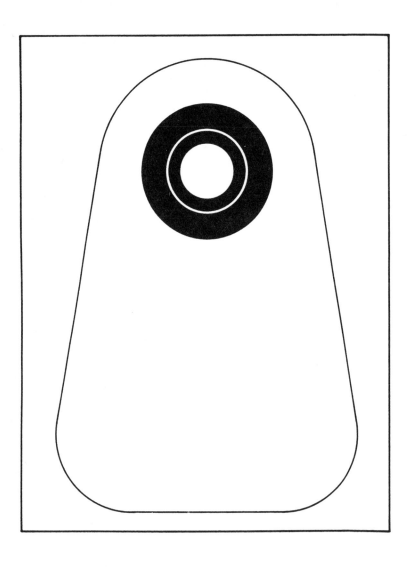

Figure 2. Closed bag or pouch with karaya ring. Also obtainable with simple adhesive flange.

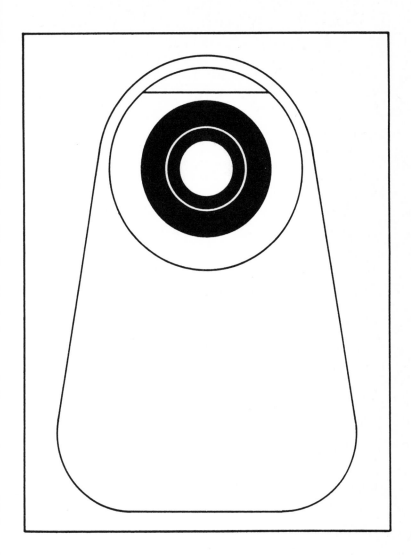

Figure 2a. Closed bag or pouch and adhesive flange incorporated to give extra security.

management as simple as possible so that eventually the colostomist does not have to be reminded unnecessarily that a stoma is a somewhat unusual physical alteration to the body image. Below, I discuss five methods of colostomy management.

1. Plastic bag, with a karaya ring which has healing properties for patients with skin problems. This bag usually has a narrow comfortable belt. There is often an efficient charcoal vent in the bag to reduce odour and gas.
2. Plastic bag which has a simple adhesive and charcoal vent. It is usually a matter of trial and error finding the right adhesive, but there are so many bags of this type on the market that it should not be difficult to find the right one.
3. Two-piece appliance which is helpful to the patient who cannot have a bag frequently removed from the skin because of excoriation, who may have arthritic hands and cannot apply the bag easily, who may not be able to move about easily, or who is partially sighted or blind.
4. Gamgee or similar dressing, with tape to hold the dressing in place, for those who cannot tolerate adhesive, and for those who choose to control the colostomy action by diet or irrigation.
5. Irrigation. This is a way of control which can be used by those who are able, with intelligence, to use the equipment for themselves, or for those who are unable to develop control and are in need of constant attention. Community nurses and stoma-care nurses find that this can help with infirm and vague patients who cannot look after themselves, but the irrigation, in these cases, has to be performed by an experienced nurse.

We will now deal with each method of management so that everyone can decide for themselves which might help them. They may find that they are quite happy with their appliance, but some find that other methods of which they were hitherto ignorant, can make life easier and happier.

1. *Karaya Ring Bag*
This is a plastic bag which various manufacturers have developed, with a belt and, in some cases, a movable flange which can be

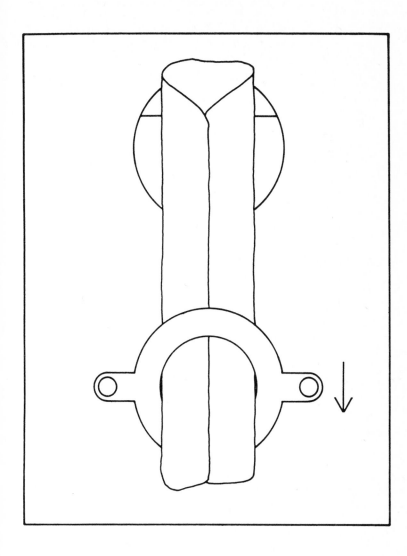

Figure 3. Closed bag with adhesive flange and removable flange for belt may be obtained with karaya ring as well as adhesive flange.

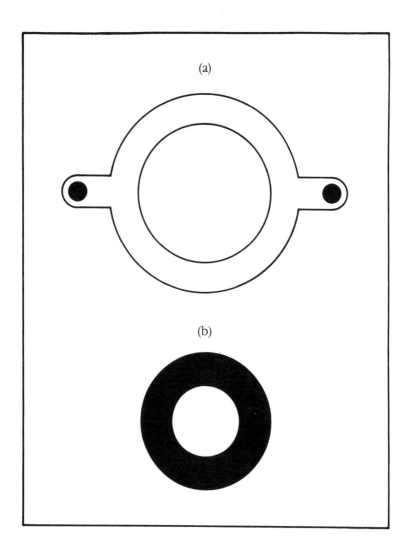

Figure 4. (a) Separate flange removed from appliance. (b) Separate karaya ring, obtainable in quantity and malleable to individual stoma size.

used to hold a dressing in place, instead of tape, when a patient does not wish to wear a bag. Some of these karaya bags also have an adhesive surround which, if the adhesive is acceptable, does give added security and support. Most types have the new improved charcoal vent which certainly does reduce odour and offensive flatus (see Figure 3).

This type of appliance can serve two purposes: it can give the patient security at night when used as a complete unit, but just the flange with a dressing can be used when the patient feels that he can safely leave off the bag (and, believe me, this is a possibility, and just needs a little courage in the security of the home, to gain confidence).

Karaya is a gum which has healing properties and has proved of immense help to those who have skin problems. Manufacturers are now producing separate karaya rings (see Figure 4a and 4b).

These rings may be moulded round the stoma. Many patients like to keep a pack of these rings so that at the first signs of the skin being sore, they can apply the healing karaya with little trouble. These rings may be used under dressings or with the ordinary plastic bag, and are very economical if used this way. Many patients find that they do not need to use the karaya bag all the time as the skin adjusts without help, so they simply keep the rings for emergencies.

2. *Plastic Bag with Simple Adhesive*
Most manufacturers produce a variety of bags with an adhesive flange which goes directly on the skin. Many skin types become accustomed to plaster in time, but one very useful hint is to expose the adhesive to the air for an hour or so before putting it on the skin, thereby reducing the sometimes drastic effect. When I use a bag, I take off the backing to the plaster so that it is exposed for several hours before putting it on, then I take the backing off the next bag to be used, even if it is six hours or more before use. This does not impair the sticking power of the plaster.

The choice of adhesives depends on individual skins and preference, so the new colostomist should not be dismayed if one or two types do not suit his or her skin. This type of bag, which is made in many sizes and lengths, may be used very successfully with the separate karaya rings, described in item 1 above.

3. *The Two-piece Appliance*

This is the ideal appliance for those who do not wish to have an adhesive removed two or three times a day, or for those who cannot easily place a bag correctly over a stoma. Those whose fingers are uncertain through arthritis or rheumatism, or who are partially-sighted or blind, or who are very old and are obliged to look after themselves without help during the day, all find the two-piece appliance an excellent method of management.

There has been an enormous improvement in this type of appliance in the past few years and the manufacturers have not relaxed their efforts to produce a really good method.

There are, of course, variations on the two-piece theme, so I will give below three of the most used types.

a.   This appliance has a pad of healing material which is placed on the skin. This pad is inset with a circular flange that snaps into the separate bag which can be changed when desired, leaving the healing material on the skin for up to three days, by which time the skin troubles should have disappeared or be well on the way to being healed.

b.   There is another type which has an adhesive flange which remains on the body during the day. Some people leave it on longer for it can be washed, and a separate bag is stuck to the flange, and removed when necessary.

c.   Yet another type has a bag which fits over a firm adhesive healing pad with a plastic flange, by means of an elastic band. The flange remains on the body for several days, and the bag with the elastic band can easily be removed. Partially sighted colostomists find this easy to manage.

4. *Non-adhesive Appliance*

There are those who cannot tolerate an adhesive of any kind. Although there are many aids, which we will look at later, even these do not help everyone; so those who are faced with this type of problem have only one way to overcome it; avoid it.

I mentioned in item 1 above that a flange with a belt, which is part of the karaya ring system, can be removed and used to hold in place a small dressing, which is adequate for the normal output of faeces, if firm. The size of dressing must be ascertained

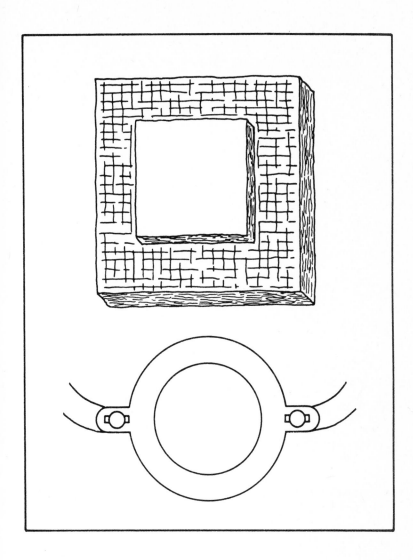

Figure 5. Pad of gamgee cut to required size with small pad of soluble tissue with removable flange and belt.

by the colostomist himself, but a 4 to 5-inch square of gamgee with a folded 2-inch square of toilet paper placed in the middle is usually sufficient. By using toilet paper, mucus is absorbed and irritation is prevented. It can easily be changed in the lavatory and replaced with another piece of toilet paper (see Figure 5).

If a patient in the early days does not have the confidence to wear a dressing at night, then a bag with a healing pad attached could be used; but the very fact that, for part of the day at least, the stoma and surrounding skin has been free of an adhesive will make the bag at night more tolerable. The healing pad, which is used in some appliances, can also be obtained separately, and may be used under a dressing to help the healing process.

Also, if a correctly balanced diet is worked out, this will help to firm the motion, making the use of a small dressing a very good method for troublesome skins. Of course, the firmer the motion, the less odour, so that does not create a problem with this method.

As time goes by, the colostomist will be able to use one of the non-irritant tapes to fix the dressing, and dispense with flange and belt.

The advanced and experienced colostomist may begin to feel that he wishes to get back to the most natural way possible of dealing with an unnatural way of disposing of the waste. One of these ways is to utilize the 'dressing' method in conjunction with diet control. A piece of wide stretch plaster, which can be doubled to about 4½ inches, if extra confidence is required, with a square of tissue in the middle, is lightly stretched across the stoma (see Figures 6a and 6b). This acts as a barrier, or muscle, and develops the stoma muscles and the storage space in the bowel. If there is no bag into which the firm motion can fall, then the body will withhold the waste until it is released by the removal of the 'barrier' or plaster. In other words, the colostomist controls the motion, not the other way round. Of course, if there is a tummy upset or a bout of flu, then bags can be used until the bowel action returns to normal. If such an upset happens, there is usually sufficient notice by added mucus and ordinary stomach ache to give time to fit a bag.

This method can be introduced slowly, if the colostomist needs confidence. Try it during the day when alone or after the normal

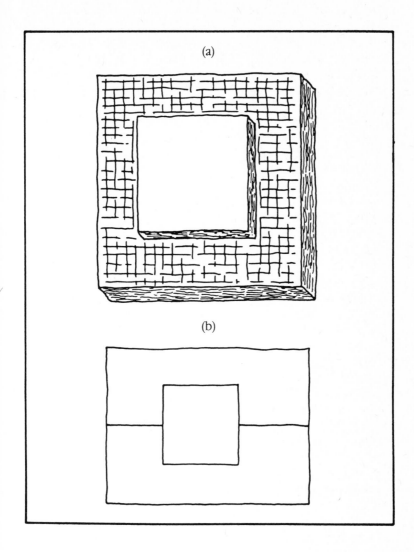

(a)

(b)

Figure 6. a) Dressing made of gamgee pad with soluble tissue for non-adhesive type of aid. b) Dressing made of two strips of plaster cut to size, with soluble tissue, for non-adhesive type of aid.

action of the day, which is usually in the morning.

Going without a bag may seem dramatic, but if the idea is acceptable, and the diet is right, then the desire to succeed is all that is needed.

5. *Irrigation*

This is sometimes known as wash-outs or colonic irrigation. It is a method by which the intestine is 'washed out' and there are certain important prerequisites. There must be suitable facilities for the irrigation to take place. The patient who is performing the irrigation must be sufficiently intelligent to be able to calculate the amount of water required, temperature and timing.

Before undertaking this type of management, the consultant must be in agreement. The instruction for irrigation must be undertaken by the stoma-care nurse or a qualified nurse attached to one of the manufacturing houses who produce the equipment.

Several appliances for irrigation are now available on the National Health Service, and the manufacturers are very helpful with their advice.

An advantage of 'wash-outs' is that a community nurse and those looking after very difficult patients may use this method to control the care of the patient, but the irrigation must be carried out by an experienced person. It is often not necessary to irrigate more than two or three times a week, but this will, of course, depend upon the diet.

Many businessmen and women like to irrigate if they are to be away from home for long periods, on business trips, conferences, flying abroad for short trips, and once they have worked out the days between irrigation, it can prove a method which does not need much thought between times. Of course, less attention has to be paid to diet which is a relief to some who have to attend luncheons and entertain customers.

Aids to Management

There are many items produced to help skin excoriation, motion control and deodorizing the faecal matter. Most of these aids are available on the National Health Service, although there are some deodorants which are not designated as being free on prescription. However, a doctor will usually prescribe such an item if it is thought necessary for the colostomist's psychological well-being. Once the GP knows the colostomist's individual problem, he is most helpful and understanding, so do not hesitate to discuss appliance and aid needs with him.

Broadly speaking, the aids to management are classified under the following headings, but the main ingredient is *Common Sense*.

— Barrier creams, skin gels and karaya powders.
— Pastes to make the bag leak-proof and to form a firm seal (not to be confused with the above creams).
— Karaya rings or squares of healing material, and flexible impregnated net.
— Pantees and net dressings to hold a dressing in place.
— Deodorants.
— Belts which firm slack muscles.

There are certain general procedures which must be observed in the interests of hygiene and personal freshness and, incidentally, personal comfort.

If there has been a motion, the bag should be emptied or changed as soon as possible. If the motion is only a small firm one which falls into the bag, or merely mucus, then it can be left, for if the bag is a good fit the odour problem will not arise and the surrounding skin will not be subjected to excessive removal of the adhesive. If a dressing or cap is worn, then the tissue covering the stoma can be removed and a fresh one inserted between the main dressing and the stoma. Any really soiled appliance or dressing should be removed as soon as possible as a protection against skin irritation and odour, especially if the motion is loose.

The stoma and surrounding skin must be well washed before applying a bag or dressing, with good plain soap, which is well rinsed away and the skin and stoma thoroughly dried. This is most important, for if soap is left on the skin the bag will not adhere properly. Too much talc, karaya powder or cream of any kind at one application will prevent the adhesive on the bag sticking properly and it will not, therefore, form a good seal. All these soothing materials should be carefully applied.

Barrier Creams and Skin Gels

After cleaning the stoma and surrounding skin, a skin gel or barrier cream should be very economically applied to about 4 inches of the surrounding skin, but not on the stoma itself. The area should be approximately the area of the adhesive on the bag so that the adhesive does not actually touch the skin, but the skin is protected by the gel. This protection is easily washed off with soap and water each time a bag or dressing is applied. The gel or cream should not be allowed to build-up by successive applications without the first application being washed off. This could cause a hard, uneven surface on the skin which has to be scraped off, and this will create further problems. These gels and creams will also protect the skin from mucus and loose faeces.

Red and Weepy Skin

Any cream or gel described here should not be applied to an excoriated skin. This needs a different treatment. The gel and cream is a preventive treatment and must be recognized as such. If used when the skin is new and unbroken, the trouble is met before it occurs.

Karaya Paste

This type of paste is produced to form a firm seal and to fill in any creases in the skin around the stoma, so that a smooth and leak-proof fit may be made. It is a somewhat coarser cream than the gel type and should be used only when the skin is wrinkled or ridged by the sutures, so that it is possible to obtain a firm fit by using this paste to fill in the gaps. These pastes should not be applied to a red or sore skin.

Excoriated Skin and Advanced Skin Problems

Sometimes small patches of skin become sore and the skin might become broken. When this occurs, an application of water-based calamine lotion might cure the irritation. If it persists, then a small piece of the healing net or pad of material, sufficient to cover the sore area, may be cut off the 4-inch piece, and placed over the soreness. The usual appliance may then be fitted over. The healing substance should be left on for two or three days. A small piece of tissue over the stoma head will help to absorb the mucus and aid the healing process. For the very red and weepy skin all

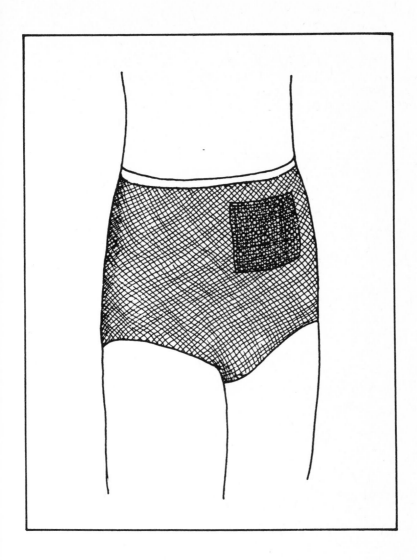

Figure 7. Net pantee with gamgee dressing or stoma cap.

round the stoma, a full piece of 4-inch healing pad or healing net should be placed. (There is a cutting guide supplied to form an even hole for the stoma.) This should be left on for at least three days, with the appliance being placed on top of the pad. The healing process will then take place without the removal of the aid.

Many patients, when the skin is very painful, find that they cannot bear any type of plastic near the stoma or stomach, especially if the broken skin extends beyond an area of 4 inches radius from the stoma. In these cases it is always better for a few days at least, to use gamgee dressings with soluble tissue against the stoma head, which can be changed quite easily when there is a motion. This dressing is held in place with a net pantee which can be obtained on prescription (see Figure 7).

However, there are the appliances described already which are made with a square of this healing material incorporated into the flange and this flange may remain on the patient for several days, the bag being changed without disturbing the healing process. Patients with a constant skin problem find it necessary to wear this type of appliance all the time, but once the skin has become tolerant, a less bulky and costly system could be used. This is where the advice of the stoma-care nurse would be helpful.

Sometimes patients find soreness develops where they have been sutured, if they have been sitting for a long time. This is where the impregnated net square of healing material can be easily moulded to the sitting area and held in place with a light and comforting dressing of gamgee. Broken skin can soon develop if not looked after in this area. Another and quick remedy for any soreness produced by pressure on the bottom is to use the ordinary water-based calamine lotion to cool the skin down. The oil-based calamine is not helpful at all. The water-based calamine soon dries and will bring great relief, as it does with sunburn, and can be easily purchased from any chemist without embarrassment. This can be of great help to those starting to drive again where there is movement while sitting. There is no need to be anxious if this slight soreness occurs long after the operation — I will have it after a long car journey even after twenty-three years. If the soreness is more than just slight then, as I have said, the impregnated square of net is the answer. The square pads are inclined to be hard and would need really softening, either in the hand or near heat, before applying to the bottom.

There are so many degrees of skin irritation that it is impossible to give a sure remedy, but there are points which should be watched:

1.   If the aperture of the bag is the wrong size, i.e. too large, allowing the faecal matter to touch a large part of the skin around the stoma, and if the motion is loose, then the skin will react. A proper fit is essential. Some bags have guide lines to help the colostomist to cut the bag to fit, or a karaya ring which can be pulled into a larger hole for the stoma. These bags are very useful, for the stoma does not remain the same size. This could be dependent upon weather, food, activity and reaction to the plastic material of the bag on the stoma skin itself.

   To increase the size of the aperture, fold the bag in half and cut round the hole to the right size. This will give an even-shaped opening.

2.   Antiseptics on the skin and stoma can cause problems and are best avoided. Pure soap and water, and a good rinsing in cool water is usually sufficient for hygiene.

3.   If the motion is loose, change the bag frequently and as soon as convenient, for several reasons. The loose motion will affect the skin, and will also cause the adhesive to lift and eventually come adrift from the skin, producing odour. So, with a loose motion, change the bag as soon as possible.

4.   See that any 'bulkers' or aids to firming the motion are properly taken. They should always be taken half an hour before food, with no liquid being taken from then until at least half an hour after the meal. If an increased liquid intake is necessary, then have more liquid at another time. Often, instructions on taking the 'bulker' on the manufacturers' labels are for many different conditions of patients, and not necessarily for colostomists. This is why I have stressed the correct way for colostomists who wish to firm their action.

Karaya Rings
The separate karaya rings are a good preventive measure if the skin

is red and slightly sore. They are flexible, can be moulded to any size of stoma and can be applied to the skin, which may be more excoriated one side of the stoma than the other, without causing an adverse reaction in the good skin. If the weather is cold and the ring seems to be solid, hold it in the palm of the hand for a while, or place it near a heater, until it is malleable, and it may then be pulled into the shape and size needed. Many colostomists use the ring round the stoma as a preventive measure in the event of a moist motion, if they tend to have problems this way. Keeping in mind the fact that stomas do change in size and the motion can change with the diet, patients who use the separate ring are taking a wise precaution, for they can be used with the normal appliance or left off if the skin does not need help.

Many bags have a karaya ring which is flexible and can be worked into the stoma size required. This is a good point to watch when choosing a bag with a karaya ring, for stomas vary slightly according to the body condition. So, it is useful to have a ring which can be moulded into the shape required, as opposed to the bag which has a predetermined size and the patient may have to have two or three different prescriptions to make a really good fit to prevent the faeces touching the skin surrounding the stoma. This is one of the reasons why, when visiting homes, one sees so many boxes of unused appliances, an unnecessary expense for the National Health Service — if the karaya ring is not flexible, the bag cannot be used on a stoma of the wrong size.

General

One very useful point to remember if using karaya rings, either attached to a bag or separately, is that used on top of a light application of skin gel, the ring will come off the skin without much problem. Sometimes, if the weather is hot and the body is perspiring, the karaya gum may melt and adhere to the skin, making a very messy surface on any possible soreness beneath the gum. The application of the gel will permit the ring or bag to be lifted without a mess or tearing of skin. If, however, the skin is already broken, the gel should not be used, but the karaya left on the skin to do its work for two or three days. After this time the karaya should be washed off with pure soap and water. If a bag is used, it should be carefully lifted and replaced with the new karaya bag.

If it is not possible to use gel on an unbroken skin, a good preventive measure is to cover the ring, either on the bag or separate ring, with a single square of surgical gauze, with a hole cut in the middle to fit to the stoma size. This will not interfere with the healing process, but will permit the karaya to be lifted more easily from the skin.

So, as a preventive measure against skin problems around the stoma, the karaya ring, with an application of skin gel, is a very good precaution before the skin problem becomes an advanced condition. However, if the skin does not give problems, do not worry about these ideas, but keep them in mind for an occasion when there may be a change in the skin texture. Prevention is better than cure anytime.

Pantees and Girdles

Many women use a pantee or girdle during the day when they are using a casual bag, dressing or a cap. The firmness of the girdle helps to keep the stomach under control and to develop the stoma muscles, so that eventually the internal storage space can be developed. The pantee is removed when the patient wishes to use the lavatory in the ordinary way, and very often the faecal matter, if reasonably firm, is ready to be released, thereby enabling it to be disposed of in the pan without further trouble. Sometimes men use a pantee girdle, especially if their wives have an old one which is not too elasticated. However a new pantee can easily be modified.

The main idea behind this type of stomach control is that it helps the muscles to develop through the system and eventually the sphincter muscle which has been removed during the operation is replaced by firmer control of the remaining end of the colon. If the stomach muscles become too relaxed and flabby, then the motion will suffer by being too slack, for it will pass through the body too quickly, apart from producing phantom pains in the rectum area and a full, bearing-down feeling.

Some larger men prefer to use the net pantee type, used to keep all kinds of surgical dressings in place. These net pantees can be used with great effect to hold a gamgee pad on the stoma, especially for those who cannot tolerate adhesives (see Figure 7).

Deodorants

One excellent, natural deodorant is parsley, which I mentioned in Chapter 1 on nutrition. If a little is taken during the day, one or two raw sprigs, many odour problems at the end of the day can be avoided. If you smoke and your partner does not, then parsley is the answer for it.

General deodorants vary considerably. The one usually employed is a liquid which is very strong and must not be permitted to touch the skin for it can cause irritation and water-blisters on the surrounding skin. One drop of this liquid is put into the bottom of the bag, rubbed into the plastic material and the bag may then be placed into position. No liquid must touch the stoma. When the faeces pass into the bag, the deodorizing effect takes place. Some bags have a small deodorizing vent at the top of the bag into which one drop of the liquid may be squeezed. This will deodorize any gas or odour which occurs in the time that the bag is in place.

Other bags have a small vent of charcoal already incorporated and if the bag is fitted properly by placing it so that the vent is near the stoma, and the adhesive flange is smoothed round the stoma from the bottom upwards, there is a reasonably good chance that there will be no odour, if the motion is not loose and watery. However, there is a variation in the quality of the charcoal vent and a patient must not be disappointed when one type of filter does not work. Once again, it must be trial and error, but eventually the right charcoal filter for you will be found — try them all if necessary. One firm of manufacturers has produced a separate charcoal filter which can be placed on a bag or dressing. I have tried it under an ordinary dressing and it is most effective. This gives great freedom to the colostomist who does not wish to be bag-oriented all day and every day.

If the plastic material used in making the bag causes the stoma to swell through heat or pressure, a piece of ordinary lavatory tissue may be folded into two thicknesses to fit the size of the individual stoma and placed on top of the stoma to protect it against the plastic. Do not be tempted to cover the stoma skin with a skin gel. The appliance can be fixed easily over this tissue, for the appliance opening should be slightly larger than the stoma.

Alternatively, the tissue may be fixed to the inside of the bag with a piece of waterproof tape so that it is opposite the stoma, avoiding contact with the plastic. This small piece of tissue will absorb the mucus and prevent it reaching the skin round the stoma, also preventing a possible cause of the stoma-head swelling.

This idea is especially helpful if the plastic rubs the stoma and causes slight bleeding, which is a common problem, and nothing to worry about, for the bleeding will soon cease if protected. If the bleeding does not cease, then contact your doctor or consultant, but this is not often necessary. The stoma skin is tender and slight bleeding does occur when cleaning, especially if dry faeces or a build-up of cream or gel has been permitted to occur. This is one of the important reasons for very careful hygiene. Always make sure that the stoma and surrounding skin is quite clean and dry before applying gel, cream or appliance. Plain soap and water cannot be beaten!

Cleaning
Many colostomists do not know how to clean the stoma in the most convenient way. Soluble paper tissues which can be put down the water closet are the most common and easy way of wiping off the stoma head without causing rubbing when cleaning.

If one is at home, then a *J-cloth*, which can be washed and mildly disinfected and rinsed, is quite helpful, for it can be cut in half and each half will last for quite a long while. The great advantage of these cloths is the ease with which they may be washed through. I would suggest that old rags, face cloths or a thicker type of material are not helpful, for this type of cloth can cause irritation to the stoma and is difficult to wash hygienically. So, this sort of cloth should be avoided. Besides, it is not very pleasant for a spouse, neighbours or even oneself to see these old rags hanging out to dry.

Disposal of Appliances
This is one of the first questions asked by new colostomists. Many older patients do not have an open fire or garden incinerator which is the most obvious way to dispose of the bags, although some of the more modern odour-proof bags do not burn easily.

When a patient is in hospital, they do not have to think of this problem, for all bags and dressings are placed in a paper disposal container and they are disposed of by the Council, or burnt in the main hospital incinerator. The usual way for a patient when returning home is to have a large pair of old scissors which can cut the bottom of the bag, releasing the contents of the bag into the lavatory pan and by flushing the pan, the bag can be 'dunked' into the clean water. The bag can then be placed on a sheet of newspaper and folded into a small square, which is then wrapped up in the newspaper and sealed off with a small piece of sellotape. Alternatively, the folded appliance may be placed into a plastic or paper bag saved from shopping expeditions, and sealed off in a small package again. It may then be placed in the ordinary waste bin. But — and this is a large BUT — do not save a large number of bags in a plastic sack and then leave the sack for the Council to dispose of. They will not do this, although most Councils permit separate bags to be mixed with rubbish. Mix the well-wrapped appliances with the ordinary waste and there will be no problem.

I have heard of some most extraordinary cases where patients did not know what to do with the used appliances. One patient used to put them down the ordinary drainage system, which meant that after a few weeks there was a blockage and a plumber had to be brought in to clean out what he called 'a load of old plastic bags'.

Another aged patient, who had only a lodger to look after her, asked him to take a plastic sack down to the river near the back garden and to 'sink it in the water'. He did not know what the bag contained, of course, or so we hope!

Yet another patient, who went on her first holiday abroad since the operation, did not know what to do with the soiled bags, and once again collected a number and she and her husband swam out to sea with a sackful between them, weighted down with stones!

Prescriptions

All patients with a stoma under pensionable age are entitled to free prescriptions and the Exemption Certificate is obtained from the Post Office. It is then presented to the GP who signs it. It is then sent to the address on the form for confirmation by the authorities.

On each prescription there is a space at the back of the form which has to be ticked if an Exemption Certificate is held, thereby entitling the patient to a free prescription. If a patient lives in an isolated region and is unable to get to a chemist, most manufacturers of appliances have a special service which will permit a prescription to be sent to them direct, and they will send the items by return of the post. The manufacturers provide a very good service and are only too happy to help. Check with the manufacturers first before sending the prescription for the first time. Their address will be found on the previous packaging or the doctor's receptionist will be able to provide the address, if it is not included in the list of *Useful Addresses* towards the end of this book.

There is no need for a long wait for a prescription to be delivered to the chemist, and if this is found to be so, then get in touch with the manufacturers. Two or three days is quite long enough to wait, although it is always wise to have a reserve supply in hand. When your current supply is finished, go on to the reserve and at the same time order your next supply.

If possible all patients should have a good supply before arriving home from hospital, even though the hospital will provide an interim supply. The doctor and community nurse should be approached at the earliest possible opportunity.

If there is an emergency, contact the manufacturers immediately or contact the stoma-care nurse if there is one attached to your local hospital, as she will have a supply of appliances and skin aids to help you out of a difficulty.

Creased and Aged Skins

Some patients find it difficult to get a really smooth fit with the appliance if the skin is creased. It has been found that if the patient can stretch out, even lean back in a chair, the skin will become smoother and the bag can be applied with greater ease. It is better to apply the lower part of the adhesive and carefully work the adhesive round to the top of the bag, making sure that there are no folds or creases in the adhesive through which there could be a leak. Also, a crease in the adhesive can cause an irritation. If the flange is too big, snip a little of the edge of the adhesive and overlap it to reduce the size and thereby avoid a leak.

Also do not stretch the skin excessively as this can cause a skin irritation when the adhesive pulls the skin together.

With this type of wrinkled skin it is even more important to have a really good fit to the stoma, otherwise the wrinkled skin will collect the faeces and then the sore skin problem can arise.

The karaya paste already mentioned is sometimes used to fill in the creases round the stoma and to create a good fit, but very old patients would need help with this.

3.

GOING ON HOLIDAY

When the trauma of the operation and having to cope with a new type of existence has been overcome, it is good to look forward to a change of environment and tempo. This may at first seem very uncertain and improbable and colostomists may be apprehensive about their ability to deal with their new way of living, in a different atmosphere.

There are several types of first holidays: day-trips, which can be arranged with convenient stops if taken by car or coach; staying at a guest house or hotel, if possible with a bathroom, but certainly hot and cold water in the bedroom; or staying with a relative who understands the problem. The important thing is for colostomists to feel confident in travelling a distance and to feel sure that they will have suitable accommodation to use when they arrive at their destination. A short, well-planned coach tour by a reputable firm is a good beginning, if a well-organized relative or friend is not available, or until the colostomist is confident enough to drive on his or her own sorties. But do not delay a holiday of some kind, for the sense of release and progress is immeasurable to the colostomist.

National Key Scheme for Toilets

From the Royal Association for Disability and Rehabilitation (RADAR) information has been received about a scheme which will provide keys for public toilets which have to be locked. While a colostomy or ileostomy is not regarded as a disability, there are of course some disabled people with stomas. Also it is sometimes convenient for an ostomist, who is not disabled, to be able to use a public toilet.

The National Key Scheme (NKS) was introduced because an increasing number of local authorities and other organizations providing public toilets felt that they had to lock their toilets either totally, or for longer hours to counter vandalism and in order to reduce the maintenance costs.

If toilets for the disabled have to be locked, local authorities and others are asked to join the NKS which involves fitting a standard lock to their toilets and making keys available to disabled people. This has now been adopted by over 110 authorities throughout the country and includes a number of seaside resorts and other areas attractive to visitors. British Rail and a number of other organizations have also joined the scheme.

The scheme is not in use everywhere, unfortunately a number of local authorities do not have any suitable toilets, and others do not have vandalism problems. However it is hoped that as many authorities as possible will participate in the distribution of keys to disabled people and that they will be widely available from Tourist Information Centres etc.

RADAR also supplies keys to those people who are unable to obtain one from their own local authority, at a cost of £2.00 to cover the price of the key and handling charges.

A list of toilets covered by the scheme is maintained by RADAR. This is regularly up-dated as more organizations join the scheme and is automatically sent out with each key that is ordered. Copies of the list can be obtained if a large stamped address envelope is sent to RADAR, Housing/Access Department. (See *Useful Addresses* at the end of this book.)

Disposal of Bags

Abroad, the routine in hotels is very much the same as in this country. Let us assume that there are no facilities to dispose of the soiled appliances. The bag is emptied and folded; put in a small paper or plastic bag, and sealed. It may then be disposed of in the waste bin, litter bin, or sani-bin, but do not stow away a large number of bags or dressings and then try to dispose of them. One at a time is the rule. If dressings are used, the disposal problem is not so difficult. The stoma cap type of dressing can be folded over on itself, and can be put in any sani-bin, or bathroom bin, for the motion will have been disposed of in the lavatory pan, and the soluble tissue can be washed down the lavatory in the ordinary way. If an elastoplast pad with tissue square against the stoma is used, then the tissue can be put down the pan and the elastoplast folded into a small square and wrapped in toilet paper or newspaper if preferred. Very often the plaster or stoma cap is not soiled so there is no hygiene problem, and the soluble tissue which is against the stoma goes down the lavatory in the usual course of events, with the faeces.

Ensuring a Supply of Appliances

If the colostomist is to be away for a number of weeks and will not be able to carry sufficient bags with him, then it is important for him to have a prescription from his local doctor, so that a further supply may be obtained. If one is travelling abroad there may be difficulty in explaining what is needed, so if the GP's prescription is carried it will help to elucidate the situation. There are, of course, many colostomists in the countries to which one may travel, so by approaching a doctor or hospital in a foreign country with a prescription from your own doctor, the dispensing of a prescription is made much easier for everyone concerned. There is an International Association with world-wide representatives, so a request for appliances is quite normal to medical personnel in other countries. However, this would apply only if one was to be away from England for more than two or three weeks, otherwise sufficient appliances can normally be carried.

If on holiday in England, always remember to get in touch with the nearest stoma-care nurse should you run out of equipment or need help. The nurses carry a stock of appliances and always provide bags of some kind in an emergency.

Customs

Many people do not realize that bags will keep well if taken out of large boxes and put in ordinary plastic freezer bags. In this way, they pack away in the luggage quite easily and can fit in between the clothes. The Customs Officers do not cause embarrassment by searching this kind of luggage, for they are fully aware of what the appliances are, but if colostomists are nervous about their equipment being exposed by the Customs, it is possible to obtain a note from the doctor, stating the function of the bags and aids. One of the advantages of using dressings and stoma caps is that there cannot be anything unusual in carrying these items. A few bags and cleaning aids should be carried in the hand-baggage in case of hold-ups or emergencies, and those who search hand-baggage at the airport ignore the appliances which may be carried. I have gone through Customs many times during my travels abroad, and have never been asked about appliances or any of the aids which I may carry. I know this is a fear that some colostomists have on their first journeys abroad, but the fear is groundless.

Insurance

I have been asked about travel insurance for colostomists. This should not cause any trouble, for unless the colostomist is under a doctor's care and has other problems to be considered, there is no reason why the ordinary insurance should be affected. Colostomists who are well-recovered are medically clear and do not regard themselves as 'patients' or 'invalids'.

Sitting Without Odour

Trains and coaches in England do not provide a problem for colostomists; I have already mentioned that in the early days I would sit in a coach or bus so that my stoma was away from the person sitting next to me, in case of an unexpected odour, but as time goes by one does not think about this happening. By sitting upright with the feet square to the floor, the possibility of the tummy being creased to a point where gas is forced out is minimized.

Air Travel

The thought of air travel is frightening to many people, be they colostomists or not, but it is very simple really. When one arrives at the airport the luggage is checked in and this will leave one free to wait for the call for one's particular flight. During this time one has passed through the check-in desk to the departure lounge where there is plenty of space, lavatories, and refreshments if required. Usually one is here for about an hour, during which time one can change the appliance, but only if necessary. When the flight call is made, the passengers move to the appropriate gate and pass on to the aircraft. By now one feels as though something is really happening, and one is on the move.

By the time one is settled on the aircraft (hand-baggage with the reserve of appliances is either at your feet or on the compartment shelf above) it is time to take-off. A meal and drink is soon forthcoming and I have never found that any aircraft food has upset me over years of air-travel. However, I always carry with me a supply of the bran-based 'slimming' tablets, previously mentioned, and I take one of these before embarking upon an unknown meal, not as a slimming aid, but I find that it helps to keep the motion normal. Also an extra tablet of *Celevac* broken up into about six pieces helps if in doubt about a foreign meal or when trying out a national dish. I have found either of these two tablets make travelling abroad less of a hazard until confidence is obtained. The tablets cut down the desire to eat foods which may be regarded with suspicion and firm any which could cause trouble. Once the first holiday has been undertaken, the whole world opens up, bringing a great sense of freedom.

Dietary Aids

A colostomist friend wanted to go down the Rhine by boat, but as she would have to share a cabin with a friend, she was very reluctant to undertake the journey. I introduced her to the plaster-dressing idea as she was very firm in her motions. She tried this for a week before her decision to undertake the journey and having found it absolutely trouble-proof, she booked up her trip for three weeks' duration. She told me that there was no problem with disposing of the plaster, which was folded and wrapped up, and the soiled soluble tissue and motion went down the lavatory, so no one knew about the colostomy. If she was uncertain about the meals she met *en route*, she took *Celevac* tablets before meals, and if she did not fancy any of the unusual cooking presented, she overcame the hunger problem by taking the bran-slimming tablets. These would carry her over until she could eat the food she knew would be acceptable to her. This colostomist was over 70 years' old when she undertook her first trip abroad after the operation.

I also used this method when I was in North Africa last year, where the food is suspect and the water even more so. By taking the bran-based tablet to cut down the appetite, and the *Celevac* tablet to firm whatever was consumed, I was helped over what could have been a disastrous diet. Despite these dangers, the journey and experience were well worthwhile.

Even in countries where one expects the same kind of food which one has been used to in the past, methods of cooking with oil and garlic and other national ingredients can prove to be troublesome. So, be prepared, but enjoy the change of scenery for there is nothing like a holiday completely away from home for someone who has thought such a break to be improbable.

Swimming and Sunbathing
Many colostomists like to swim and sunbathe. The type of swim suits now available in shops are not very suitable for the briefs are very brief and do not come up high enough to cover a small casual bag or dressing. I have searched for an attractive 'cover-all' costume and have found that one or two good manufacturers make tunic-type costumes with separate pants. These costumes are expensive but last for a long time and answer all requirements. I have for many years worn my husband's cast-off trunks which I use with a separate top for a quiet garden sunbathe. For men with a colostomy or ileostomy it is difficult to find trunks which reach the waist, especially if the person concerned is inclined to be chubby.

However, the journal of the Ileostomy Association (see *Useful Addresses*) has mentioned that there is a company making trunks which have an eleven-inch rise from the crotch to the waist and this would be suitable for ostomists up to about 5 ft 11 ins to

6 ft tall. So for big ladies and chubby gentlemen it might be helpful to find out more about the swimwear made by Pegasus.

Salt & Son Ltd., whose address is under *Useful Addresses* at the end of this book, are now supplying *Anita* swimwear, details of which may be obtained from them if you send a stamped addressed envelope. Also CaSal of Downton are offering swimwear for ostomists; some items are even made to measure. (See *Useful Addresses*.) A stamped addressed envelope is required for brochure and sample fabrics.

4.

PERSONAL RELATIONSHIPS

When all the practical approaches to a colostomy by way of diet, appliances and aids have been explored, there always remains the unasked questions about personal relationships, marital compatibility and the acceptance of the new way of life by the partner in a close relationship, be it man or woman.

Just as there are many forms of diet and appliances, the spectrum of personal attitudes and acceptance of the operation is very wide. Some colostomists are wonderfully philosophical, prepared to adjust and are very thankful for the opportunity to be alive and useful, and each new obstacle overcome gives a great sense of achievement. There are those who after many months, or even years, still cannot but feel revulsion towards themselves and everything to do with the operation, and if these colostomists have a spouse or partner, their attitude will of course affect that partner, making a happy relationship very difficult. Some of these patients will withdraw from contact with the outside world, while others will go to the other extreme and tell everyone about their problems.

Of course the operation should be discussed with a spouse or partner at the time of the surgery, and it is very often at this time that a well-recovered colostomist can be called upon to help the partner or relative through this very difficult period when the person concerned wonders how he or she can possibly cope with the situation when the patient returns home. A talk with a vintage colostomist who has a well-balanced and healthy attitude to life and sex, can prevent many a potentially difficult situation developing, such as the break-up of a marriage or partnership.

When visiting patients in a pre-operative situation, I have been asked many questions about swimming, playing tennis, cycling, smoking, drinking and eating, but it is very often only when patients return home to the quiet of their own environment that the questions about their marital life and personal relationship with their partner comes to the fore. This is a very sensitive area, for what can be discussed quite freely with one patient may cause extreme embarrassment to another, and only a very careful conversation may produce a picture of that patient's attitude to the relationship with his or her spouse or partner.

Since I started this book I have seen many old friends and colleagues in order to recapitulate on their progress and quality of life. I am most grateful to those who have been so willing to talk, giving their permission to mention their problems, for so little information in this field is available. I feel that in this vast area it is the practical experience of others that will help with some of the problems a new and very green colostomist encounters, apart from making the new colostomist realize quite early on that others have gone through similar relationship problems.

SPOD

There is an association of highly qualified and specialized workers who, under the chairmanship of Dr Wendy Greengross, can arrange for an appointment or advice to be submitted by letter, if the patient so prefers. This organization is called SPOD (Sexual and Personal Relationships of the Disabled). The address is included in the list of *Useful Addresses* and while those with colostomies do not regard themselves as disabled, undoubtedly many need help from people who are practical and have experience in handling these delicate problems.

The outlook of both the public and professional workers at

the time of the initial research by SPOD amounted to a denial of sexuality among disabled people and viewed them as sexless. Workers in the caring professions were neither trained nor encouraged to deal with such problems and it was evident that a gap in social provision existed; so in the mid-1975 period SPOD went into the active field. The aims of SPOD are formulated below.

1. Stimulate public and professional awareness of sexual needs and difficulties among disabled people and of measures which may alleviate their problems in this respect.
2. Provide a centre for the collection and dissemination of information in this field, for disabled people themselves and for those concerned in their welfare.
3. Provide an advisory referral service for disabled clients, therapists, counsellors and educators.
4. Arrange for the training of those working among the disabled in the sexual aspects of disability.

The implementation of measures to meet these aims has been nation-wide and development has been rapid. There are workers and researchers as well as the patients themselves in five continents making contact with the SPOD Committee and it is good to know that Great Britain is now in the fore-front of those countries with a growing interest in the sexual and personal relationship side of handicap.

SPOD Committee now provides:

1. Factual information and advice.
2. Referral of clients for personal counselling.
3. Collaboration and advice on the planning of study days, symposia and conferences, and the provision of speakers if required.
4. Articles and papers for the public and professional press, house journals etc.
5. Collaboration in any bona fide venture for the support or assistance of handicapped people in sexual difficulty.

Other publications have been produced, notably the following books by members of SPOD Committee:

— *Entitled to Love* by Dr Wendy Greengross, published by the National Marriage Guidance Council, in association with the National Fund, 1976.

— *Handicapped Married Couples* by Dr Michael and Ann Craft, published by Routledge and Kegan Paul, 1979.

— *Sex and Spina Bifida* by W.F.R. Stewart, published in co-operation with SPOD.

There is a series of SPOD Advisory Leaflets on specific groups of problems and their solutions available on application to the SPOD address in *Useful Addresses* at the end of this book.

The Ileostomy Association

The Ileostomy Association produces *Ileostomy Quarterly*, a journal which is sent to every member. An associate membership of I.A. may be obtained by a colostomist and the journal is sent to them as associates of the Association. The subscription is very modest. This journal contains articles of interest, news and views, and advertisements of manufacturers' latest products. Other literature is also available on application to the new I.A. Headquarters (see *Useful Addresses*).

The Ileostomy Association also has a Personal Relationship Advisory Service to which a colostomist may write, but of course this service is more for ileostomists. The Association also organizes trials for the Department of Health and Social Security and companies who sell or produce appliances and aids, many of which are suitable for both the colostomist and the ileostomist.

Many people who have a relationship problem think theirs is the only one and that it is unique, but this is seldom the case, and it is comforting to feel that there is a source to which one can write for advice. I know from conversations with colostomists that their own particular problems cause embarrassment, so with the approval of the colleagues concerned I would like to tell you of some of the cases which can arise and the way in which they have been handled, either by the colostomist or by advisers.

A Typical Problem

SPOD was born out of the realization that there was no training in personal problems within the caring professions. I can give you one very recent instance indicating that this is still found to be so. I had visited an attractive fifty-year-old patient in hospital whose operation seemed to be quite satisfactory and she asked me to visit her at home. After a week she telephoned me to say she was at home and was very unhappy. I took with me for this visit a very young-looking seventy-year-old friend who is a colostomist as well as having a mastectomy, and blessed with a delicious sense of humour. When we arrived we found that the patient and her husband were very distressed because they had been told when they asked about their sex-life that at fifty they would have to forget all about 'that kind of thing'. My seventy-year-old friend said 'Well, I don't know about you, but twice a week is just about right for me.' The rest of the visit was hilarious, but this is a situation which should never have arisen and the question of marital life after a colostomy should have been handled more sensitively. If the couple needed anything more than encouragement, then they should have been referred to those who are trained, such as those in SPOD, or to a well-recovered colostomist who had probably experienced this situation.

A Colostomist Way of Life
At the beginning of this book I mentioned in the definition of colostomy and ileostomy that an ileostomy was usually performed on younger people, while the colostomy was more of an older persons's operation. This is statistically so, but in practice there are of course exceptions. One of the youngest colostomists I have met is an eight-month-old-girl and there is another young person who will shortly be eighteen years of age who has progressed through babyhood, growing-up and all the rigours of school-life, which is never easy for a sensitive individual. Yet this young colostomist's attitude of mind and strength of character has overcome the disappointments of not being as other young people,not having to give a thought to physical restrictions. Life is very full, but of course the difficulties up to now must have created problems for the young colostomist and the unfailing help of the parents, for whom one must have the utmost admiration, cannot be overvalued. The parents and the young colostomist have given me permission to tell the story of this wonderful family in the hope that it will encourage others — either the child

colostomist or the parents — who may find themselves in this situation.

The day after our third child was born I tried to breast-feed him, but he was refusing and vomiting. The nurse took him back to the nursery and I was not allowed to feed him until the following day. On the Wednesday following his birth we had the same performance only this time he was straining to open his bowels. Once again he was taken back to his nursery where the doctor and the nursery staff kept an eye on him. The paediatrician decided to X-ray, but at the end of ten days we were allowed to go home. He was discharged as a normal baby and his weight was beginning to increase after a severe drop.

Five days later he became lethargic over his feed and just wanted to sleep. However, as he was not passing urine or stools, I took him to the doctor who said that the baby would probably need an operation, but prescribed medicine. However, at six weeks he would not take feeds and was vomiting repeatedly and had no use of the bowels. I rushed him to the doctor again, after which my husband and I drove him to the hospital that same evening. We waited while tests were made and the doctor told us that the baby was very ill indeed. He spent his first Christmas in hospital after which it was decided in January to perform an emergency operation, and to save him he had a colostomy.

My husband and I did not really know what this would entail, but we soon had to find out. That winter was one of the worst on record, taking three hours to do a thirty-minute journey to the hospital. When we saw him lying so helpless with tubes everywhere we wondered if we had done the right thing in agreeing to this kind of operation. This was the first of many operations when he had to fight for his life.

Gradually, he started to improve and about two weeks later I was asked if I would like to feed him. I has been expressing milk to take it to the hospital, but had not actually fed him for several weeks.

For the first time I saw his tummy and nearly died on the spot. In those days there were not any baby bags suitable so he had to wear a layer of gamgee tissue covered with bandages. Naturally, being so young he had no control at all so his clothes were being continually soiled. At five months old he was allowed home to the delight of the family, and at last he was putting on weight, and was nearly seven pounds, which was two and a half pounds less than his birth weight.

The first years were the most troublesome. His tummy was so scarred, no dressing or adhesive would stick, so his dressings had to be constantly changed as well as having his nappies changed, which meant several changes during the night.

For four years he spent nearly as much time in hospital as at home, including his first and second birthdays. It was about this time that I was given the opportunity to take him to Lourdes. An organization from our Church had heard of his illness and provided the money for us to go. My husband and friends were wonderful in their help with our other children to allow me to go with him to Lourdes. We left by coach for Victoria and continued the journey by train, boat and train. It was a long and tiring journey and he needed his tummy seen to about twelve times during that time. I was exhausted when we arrived, but he wanted to go outside to play football. One thing which has amazed people is that, despite his disability, he has never in any way let it stop him behaving and playing like other children.

Had he been an only child, perhaps we would not have let him do some of the things which we just took for granted with other children. He bathed in the Holy Baths while I just hoped and prayed — yet seeing so many others in a far worse state than his, I suddenly realized that we were lucky to have a child who was at least mentally fit.

Before we left England we had been told that he would have to go to a special school, so this was our worry when we returned home. When I met the headmistress of the school where our other children were I said, 'What will happen to him?' and she reassured us that she would take him at that school and would see to him whenever necessary during the day. This was our miracle for we knew that he would now have the same attention as our other children and the same opportunities. The headmistress took him into her office three or four times during the school hours to see to his dressings.

He has always taken part in all activities, apart from swimming, and was a strong member of the school football team. He had boundless energy on and off the pitch, and still has. Soon after he started senior school it was decided he should go to Great Ormond Street Hospital in London. This stay included his twelfth birthday, and by this time he had had fourteen operations. Unfortunately tests proved that it would not be possible to reverse the colostomy and he was almost relieved that he would not have to have another operation. Since then appliances have improved so that he can now wear a bag with stomahesive. He is just starting his last year in the sixth form at school and he is a prefect. He has won his colours for cross-country running, representing his school in county events. He plays squash, cricket and tennis and his advice to other young ostomists is to have a go and join in as much as possible. As parents we are grateful to have had the opportunity to see him grow into a young man who would not give in despite everything. His will-power, and determination have helped him in many a crisis and as we look at our fine children, we realize that they all have had something to offer.

I have quoted this moving story at length because I feel that it has a message for everyone, whatever their age: for the young ostomist who is reserved about the stoma; for the relatives who wonder how they can cope; and for the caring and supportive professions who can do just that little more, like the headmistress in this case, for she gave him an educational future, and those who can study the needs of an ostomist just a little more deeply, so that the patient becomes a healthy and useful member of society.

Forming Relationships

Of course this is not the end of their story, for this young person will be wishing to form a relationship with someone as time goes by, and will need all the careful help and thought of older colostomists who may have had to cope with personal and sexual problems; for from whom else is help forthcoming, but those who have already coped as colostomists?

One of the most sound pieces of advice I received in my early days as a colostomist was to establish quite early on in a relationship, but not immediately, that I had a colostomy, to make light of it and then ignore it in everything else that I did in everyday things, showing the non-colostomist friend that life does go on and that the stoma can be forgotten in most circumstances.

The non-colostomist will, in all probability, accept the situation, but if not, then the position has been made clear without unnecessary hurt occurring later on in the relationship. It is largely ignorance of what a colostomy is and how it functions which may cause rejection by a non-colostomist, but it is up to colostomists to show that they are perfectly normal in every other way, and probably a good deal healthier than most.

When the colostomist is young and unmarried, it is bound to be more difficult to establish a relationship with someone if the colostomist is reluctant to tell the new and intended partner about the stoma. If there is a real horror of mentioning it to the friend, then carry on for a while, do all the natural and normal things, proving to oneself and the world that one is capable of having a normal relationship, then when sufficient confidence is gained, the right moment will present itself. By then, if the relationship is going to be good, this difference in your physical self will not matter so very much.

I recall to mind a young girl I met in hospital who had a urostomy and was in the process of being given a colostomy. She and her fiancé, whom I met, were planning on getting married six months hence, in the spring. The attitude of mind of both these young people was right — to meet anything which may come to them in their life together.

Dispelling Ignorance
When a somewhat older and married patient has the operation, it is most important for the partner to the relationship to be put in the picture by the surgeon, then have the practicalities of management explained by the stoma-care nurse and someone competent to give advice on the personal relationship approach, possibly by a well-recovered colostomist, for this advice will make all the difference to the patient's return home and the attitude of the non-colostomist. If the patient is a woman, the husband or partner should be made aware of the physical capabilities of the colostomist, who has recently returned home for if there is understanding on the partner's side, the adjustment to normal marital life is assisted beyond expectations. One of the underlying fears of a husband or wife is that they will be unable to cope with the physical side of their relationship. There is always the fear of being rejected by their partner and, if the motion is loose, the fear of being unacceptable is very great and very real.

Ignorance in any case causes anxiety and one twenty-three-year-old patient told me that she thought she was stitched up 'thereabouts'. She wanted children and the operation seemed to her to be the end of her marriage. There is also the fear a woman has that she will be hurt or damaged in some way during intercourse. Imagine what it means to have the worry of the possibility of an 'accident' at the same time as the fear of damage to oneself.

The Problems of Women

Women seem to be far more concerned with the possibility of the loss of their partner through the colostomy than a man may be, for in the early days odour, gas and appliances all seem to be too much to cope with as well as love-making. If a woman cannot overcome the thought of discomfort through intercourse, and if she lacks confidence in there being no action while making love, then the whole effort could be disastrous.

A woman who has become a well-recovered colostomist should have no difficulty with intercourse. The vagina may be a little tight at first, and apprehension can cause this tightness to be increased, but a relaxed woman should have no problem. With the tender and careful help of the partner, life should prove to be fulfilling and she can then concentrate on receiving and giving happiness. In the early period, when confidence is lacking and it is felt that a bag should be worn all the time, if intercourse seems likely, it is essential that the bag is empty and flat. A bag-cover may be worn if desired, but a much better idea is to fold the bag up and fix it with a small piece of water-proof plaster, so that it can be forgotten and will not look too obvious.

If there is sufficient confidence in the daily motions so that the colostomist does not feel that there will be a motion during intercourse, a stoma cap or dressing made of plaster, described in Chapter 2 on appliances, is quite adequate and hardly noticeable to the partner or the colostomist. It only takes two or three occasions using this method for complete confidence to develop. This is where knowledge of the daily diet and the outcome is so important, but it would seem that there is seldom a motion when intercourse actually takes place. Some women rely upon codeine phosphate or similar drugs taken half an hour or so before love-making — it does not matter if intercourse does not take place as these drugs will not do any harm — but this is not a really necessary aid if the motion is normal and firm. I have not known there to be a sudden rush of uncontrollable faeces during intercourse in all the years of discussing this problem with colostomists and it has never happened to me — so take heart.

Many colostomists fear that the bag will burst with pressure upon the body, but if the bag is clear of flatus when love-making starts, it is unlikely that the bag would be so full as to cause any awareness of it being upon the body and it certainly would not burst.

In a stable relationship the convalescent period does not usually present much difficulty, for while the physical side is very important in any partnership, there is much love and caring which can be demonstrated by other means. Very often new ideas and experimentation open up an entirely new and satisfying area and a marriage which was becoming rather stale before the operation, if patience is observed for a few months, can become refreshed and re-energized. If in the first months intercourse is painful, then a change of position or role in the activity can help.

I would like to tell of a youngish colostomist I have known for many years whom I contacted about this book, and she told me of her experiences, which I quote in her own words.

> When I first came out of hospital nothing was mentioned on the subject of sex at all, and at that time I did not feel like asking anyway. It was certainly a long time before I thought of any sex as in fact I was terrified of the idea, not knowing if I could cause any damage. My husband was very patient over this time and tried to get me to overcome this fear, and around eight months later I thought it only fair to him that I had to try. Things were a little strained at first owing to this fear of damage, but gradually it was overcome, perhaps a few different positions from before, so we were happy and I think other people would be the same if only they knew it would be all right. It does help, of course, when you have a helpful and considerate husband. This does not make compulsive reading and it is not much, but it may help someone.

This lady is attractive, smartly dressed and in every way a desirable person, and I think her story is typical of so many neither young nor old female colostomists, and her experience *is* compulsive reading to the many who do not know.

Of course not all patients leave hospital to return to a happy environment. Many, because they live alone, do not go out as much as they should. This type of patient tends to be in the older age range and it is then that they need to have the full support of the caring professions. The stoma-care nurse, the community nurses and health visitors, and the Home Help Service can all play a part in building a relationship with the outside world helping to restore the right attitude of mind to enable the colostomist to come to terms with the business of living.

There are those of course who return to a disrupted marriage and a hopeless sense of floundering around with no future in view, and yet there has to be an end or solution somewhere, for that is life. Once again, I quote from the actual words of one such colostomist.

> My operation was very sudden and there had been no warning that I would end up with a colostomy. From the onset of investigations to returning home with a stoma was some eight weeks. I was terrified of all physical contact and this was not helped by a husband who was impatient and without understanding of the most simple stoma function, like needing the bathroom in order to keep oneself clean. Maybe the fact that the marriage was unhappy owing to his infidelity did not help. He left the house twelve weeks after I returned home and my doctor told me that my husband has been frightened of the responsibility of looking after an invalid for life!
>
> There was a divorce and my two teenage children were marvellous. I finished their education and they now have their own young families.
>
> As you know, I have remarried, having lived with my second husband for five years, for I had to be sure and I could not take the risk of rejection again. My life has been completely fulfilled in every way, sexually, intellectually and in everyday activities, for mine is a loving man.

This colostomist is a great person of some sixty years of age, who has overcome a marriage that broke up, finally, through the operation, worked in a full-time professional job, brought up a family and still had time to remarry into a good relationship, and she told me that her physical life had never been better.

Another colostomist told me that after her operation she and her husband talked over the subject of intercourse and it was decided that because he was getting on towards 60 years old and had a tummy, they should try a different position, so she the colostomist, agreed that it might be better for him. She had not told him in all the years of their marriage that she was seven years older than her husband and she has kept her secret. And they still enjoy life some ten years after her operation.

An old friend of mine who is an inveterate long-distance traveller, had a colostomy in 1977. She and her female companion of many years and over many journeys, set off one year after the operation to rediscover over four months places previously visited in Europe. They have since ventured into far distant places and over much longer periods.

Partner's Problems

There are, of course, those who do not adjust to the new life of a colostomist, be it the colostomist himself or the partner; such as the colostomist who had been so unhappy with home life that she had two breakdowns after her return from hospital, each time requiring admission to hospital. I was asked to visit her at home by the hospital and she also telephoned me desperately from home asking for an immediate call.

When I arrived I was met by a charming lady, well-dressed and very apologetic for asking me to come in through the kitchen door, because her husband had decided to perform his exercises in the hallway when he heard my car arrive. This spouse could not bear, among other problems, to have his wife given more attention than himself and she was desperate in case she had to return to hospital as the only escape from her husband's problems. This colostomist could have been a completely well-adjusted person had outside pressures not taken over. As a colostomist she was well-recovered and able to cope with the management, but it was not her problem but her husband's.

Similarly, there is the case where the husband could not bear to hear or see anything to do with the operation, appliances or literature about the house. The wife did not know what to do with her 'bits and pieces' as she called them. With a little help and thought she realized that she could keep everything out of sight and after explaining to her that sexual intercourse was quite possible in the ordinary course of events and nothing to worry about if approached with common sense and her doctor's approval, the home situation improved. She had returned home two years previously to an isolated village and because her husband could not accept the operation, appliances, regular return visits to the clinic and the daily care needed with a stoma, there had been no physical contact and the marriage had become very tense. When she kept the bags and 'bits and pieces' out of sight and arranged for a friend to drive her to the clinic in the hospital, she was able to approach her husband with confidence and the tension began to disappear slowly.

Consideration for Others

Of course, there is the colostomist who returns home and expects everyone — husband, doctors and relatives — to regard her as an invalid. Unless the consultant and GP feel that the colostomist needs special treatment, there is absolutely no reason why this should be so. Certainly colostomists need a bathroom and lavatory for a certain amount of time every day, but not necessarily for much longer than non-colostomists, unless they irrigate the colon, which can be done when the bathroom is not needed by other members of the family, at a time when the colostomist can relax during the process. The physical capabilities return as strength returns to the patient, but the convalescent period should be limited to only a few weeks, depending upon the attitude of the patient. In other words, the sooner patients can look after themselves, clear up the bathroom and dispose of their appliances, the better for the morale of all concerned. Eventually, if patients have to do this for themselves, the sooner they will contrive methods of operation to suit their households.

Some patients rely upon husband, relatives and their helpers too much to look after the unpleasant side of having a colostomy, and if it is a husband who is being asked to deal with this aspect, the more likelihood there is of relationship problems developing. If the relationship is already strained, then the colostomist is simply asking for more problems. So, be independent, accept the stoma and convince everyone else that it is just another way of living which does not interfere with anyone else.

The Problems of Men

The male approach to a colostomy or an ileostomy is somewhat different from that of the female. However, young males will not vary too much, for they will all have the problem of personal relationships with other young unmarried people who do not have a stoma and they will tend to be reserved about telling a new friend of their operation. Thus, the previous comments relating to females could be looked at from the male angle. The consultant's views on the individual colostomist is most important and the young colostomist should not be shy about asking for the surgeon's advice when he returns for check-ups.

If there is difficulty in obtaining and maintaining an erection, this could be a temporary anxiety problem, and professional advice could help to alleviate the tension. However, to the older male colostomist who may already have a family, intercourse is more for pleasure, the natural release of tension and the giving one to another, rather than procreation — so some of the problems, often temporary and psychological, do not take on such large proportions.

Some of the factors are physical and the consultant can be of help to determine whether the problem is physical or psychological. There are, of course, those who feel uncertain about their capabilities and therefore find excuses for not trying. If the management, odour, flatus and consistency of faeces is understood and covered by all the help available the male colostomist just needs the loving consideration of the partner, for in the early stages it could be detrimental to attempt intercourse before the colostomist is feeling strong enough physically, and this could affect the psychological recovery if there is a failure.

One colostomist, who was approaching the age of sixty-four when the operation was performed, told me his very engaging story, which will illustrate this point. When he returned home, his wife had prepared the spare room with all the necessary empty cupboards for his 'equipment'. After some three weeks, during which time he was gradually feeling stronger and learning to cope with the everyday mechanics of a colostomy, his wife gently suggested that he might like to return to their bedroom. He felt somewhat dismayed at what this would mean, for it was still early days to overcome the shock and depression of a major operation. He suggested, equally gently, that he should be given a little more time.

Before his stay in hospital he had always got up first to make the early morning tea, but now his wife performed this chore. One morning, a little while later, his wife brought in the tea as usual and quietly slipped into bed, showing him that as a man he was still necessary to her. This was what he needed at this point, a little push to bring him out of the period of shock and into a great deal of love. This couple are a lively and energetic pair, taking an interest in everything that is going on around them. He will be seventy years old this year.

In the early days medication is often taken and this can cause a slowing down of responses. The ordinary 'bulkers' do not come into this category, for they can help the psychological fear of a loose motion. Alcohol can also have a disastrous effect upon the output, usually making the faeces very watery and unpredictable if taken in regular and large amounts. Beer is a great enemy of the male colostomy patient, if taken daily in several pints. The odd shandy or half-pint is all right, but the food should be of a non-loosening variety if drink is taken within an hour of eating. Many men turn to alcohol when they find that they cannot obtain or maintain an erection in the early days of convalescence. This will make all the ideas on management more difficult, for alcohol is very loosening and needs to be well observed, apart from the health hazards. It is well known that alcohol can affect a non-colostomist in reducing the sexual urge, so one can imagine how much more this will be so in the case of the convalescent colostomist.

Male colostomists may feel totally inadequate if there is one failure in intercourse which can set off a series of psychological problems, and the colostomist may even blame the operation for this failure. Everyone at sometime or another has a failure, either in performance or intenseness through over-tiredness or ill-health. A partner is likely to have had this occur before the operation, so she will be understanding if it occurs after a major operation. It is the partner's encouragement at this time that will bring the male colostomist through to a normal enjoyment of life.

One wife of a fifty-year-old male colostomist has told me of her marvellous experience. She was his second wife, some twelve years younger, and they had one child, when he developed symptoms which meant investigations. The operation for a colostomy was performed and he returned home with a very troublesome action. He had to give up his job as a senior engineer and, after much correspondence with various manufacturers of appliances trying to find a suitable type for himself (which was very difficult some twelve years ago as there was little choice and information), he was offered a consultancy with such a firm of manufacturers.

One of his difficulties was that, although he could obtain an erection, he could not maintain this long enough to help his wife, and this made him feel very inadequate. He was very distressed and, in a relationship where there was much love, they experimented with new ideas and positions. As the wife has told me, their sexual life developed beyond expectations and they have both told me that it is better than before the operation. One day she was not feeling too well, so went to her doctor, thinking that she had been overworking, as she also had to take a job because of her husband's reduced income. The doctor said with astonishment that she was pregnant, much to the joy of them both. Although somewhat a surprise to a fifty-plus colostomist who has been given to understand that it was not possible, their son, now over ten, is a great character and comfort to them.

Another much younger wife told me that she discovered that she was pregnant about three years after her husband had a colostomy, and because he was over fifty years old they decided he should have a vasectomy operation for he did not want her to be left later on in life with young children. This did not affect his sexual ability, either.

Every Partnership is Different

When considering the personal and sexual relationships of ostomists and indeed any person who might be thought of as disabled, it must be realized that each partnership is unique. There are many who do not feel that they wish to tie another person to them for life, so undertake an association which, in many cases, proves to be long and loving. One attractive woman of thirty-nine underwent all the usual fears of intercourse and, as she was a divorcee when she had the operation, found it very difficult to form a relationship with anyone. In fact, she never got round to telling any of her early possible friends of the stoma, and consequently they thought she was emotionally cold. After some six years she met a very gentle kind man and together they had many outings and sorties to the coast, where they would sunbathe and swim. Still she had not told him of the stoma. After some months he asked her to marry him, but explained that he was not very good on the physical scene, and it was at this point that she told him quite easily and naturally that she had a colostomy. He was amazed to think that there could be any physical difference in her of which he had no inkling, and their mutual problems proved the ideal mixture for this partnership.

Another old friend, who had in the thirties been a well-known West End actor, came to me on behalf of a friend of his who had also been on the stage. This friend had recently lost his life-long companion and was now shattered to be told that he was to have a colostomy. This was a very difficult case, for little comfort could be given apart from putting him in touch with a male colostomist of a similar temperament to give him a little confidence to undertake the operation, for as he said, 'who wants a middle-aged homosexual with a colostomy?' This patient suffered severe depression and would have been the right patient to have contact with SPOD had it then been in action.

Another case which has proved to be not unusual is that of the colostomist who was the owner of a chain of hotels. When he returned home he found that his wife could not cope with the situation. By virtue of his business he had easy access to alcohol and had been an alcoholic when he entered hospital, but had not told any of the hospital staff. His sexual life was unsatisfactory and his wife ignored him, and the operation resulted after a few months in her leaving him. He reacted by going on a mammoth binge. If this alcoholic patient had told the hospital staff when he went into hospital, much trouble and anxiety could have been avoided and the proper advice would have been given then to help this disease. He admits this and realizes that he must have given the staff much trouble when help would have been forthcoming had they known. Indeed, everyone in the caring professions would have given him support to overcome the problem.

There is much joy to be obtained from life and at most times all people have to adjust to different situations and ideas. However, there is nearly always someone who can come forward with an answer or helpful suggestion. For the colostomist or ileostomist it is usually someone who has had a stoma who can see and feel the anxiety and misery of a personal relationship which is going wrong. The caring professions are wonderful in their help with all the practicalities and nursing skills, but the mental anxieties and worries which may occur after the operation are another thing entirely. I understand that more training is being considered for the back-up teams in the field of sexual and personal relationships, and this additional insight and knowledge by the non-colostomist cannot be undertaken too soon. Even after twenty-three years of work with colostomists I realize that every new ostomist I meet is a new challenge and, above all, is an individual who has to have a *new concept of living.*

USEFUL ADDRESSES

Help and Advice

Age Concern, Bedford House, Pitcairn Road, Mitcham, Surrey. Always useful to contact about transport and other domestic problems. Local representatives in most areas.

British Chiropractors' Association, 5 First Avenue, Chelmsford, Essex. Tel. 0245 53078. The Association will provide list of qualified Manipulative Practitioners.

Community Nurses. Contact is made through your doctor, stoma-care nurse, or health visitor.

The Journal of the Ileostomy Association, Amblehurst House, Chobham, Woking, Surrey. Tel. 099 05 8277. Journal gives up-to-date information and many interesting articles.

In Touch. Free magazine for stoma patients printed by Searle Medical, Freepost P.O. Box 88, Lane End Road, High Wycombe. Will provide list of stoma-care nurses throughout the country.

Medical Social Worker. Contact through Social Services Department. Any problems may be discussed with these experienced people, who will know where help is to be obtained.

Osteopaths. The British Naturopathic and Osteopathic Association

6 Netherhall Gardens, London NW3 Tel. 01-435 7830. A list of qualified practitioners will be provided.

Royal College of Nursing, Cavendish Square, London, W1. Tel. 01-409 3333. For list of Stoma Care Nurses throughout the country.

SPOD Sexual and Personal Relationships of the Disabled 286 Camden Road, London N7 OBJ. Tel. 01-607 8851.

National Key Scheme, Royal Association for Disability & Rehabilitation, (RADAR) 25 Mortimer Street, London, W1N 8AB, Tel. 01-637 5400.

Manufacturers and Suppliers of Appliances and Aids

Most of the firms mentioned below provide the appliances and aids mentioned in this book. If in doubt, write to the company concerned to see if they offer a prescription dispensing service, and an advisory stoma-care unit, and ask for details of any items which interest you.

Abbott Laboratories Ltd., Queenborough, Kent ME11 5EL. Tel. Sheerness 3371. Appliances, karaya aids, stoma cap, irrigation equipment.

CaSal, Parsonage Farm House, Barford Lane, Downton, Salisbury, Wilts SP5 3PZ. Swimwear.

Coloplast Ltd., Somersham Road, St Ives, Huntingdon, Cambs PE17 4LN. Tel. St Ives 62600. Appliances and aids.

Downs Surgical Ltd., Church Path, Mitcham, Surrey CR4 3UE, Tel. 01-640 3422 and 01-648 6291. Appliances and karaya aids.

Eschmann Bros & Walsh Ltd., Peter Road, Lancing, W. Sussex BN15 8TJ. Tel. Freephone 3128. Appliances and karaya aids.

Squibb Surgicare Ltd., 141-149 Staines Road, Hounslow, Greater London TW3 3JB. Tel. 01-572 7442. Stomahesive healing pads and appliances with healing pads incorporated.

Searle Medical Products, P.O. Box 88, Lane End Road, High Wycombe, Bucks HP12 4HL. Tel. High Wycombe 21124. *In Touch* magazine sent free on request. Appliances, aids and deodorant liquid.

Simpla Plactics Ltd., Phoenix Estate, Caerphilly Road, Cardiff, CF4 4XG. Tel. Cardiff 62100. Appliances, aids, liquid deodorant.

Salt & Son Ltd., 220 Corporation Street, Birmingham B4 6QR.

Tel. 021-233 1038. Appliances and aids.

Smith & Nephew: Bessemer Road, Welwyn Garden City, Hertfordshire AL7 1HF. Tel. Welwyn Garden City 25151. Elastoplast elastic adhesive bandage and Jelonet healing squares.

Chas F. Thackray Ltd., Box 171, Park Street, Leeds LS1 1RG. Tel. Leeds 42321. The Care Centre, 47 Great George Street, Leeds, LS1 3BB. Tel. Leeds 442329. Appliances and aids.

Thames Valley Medical Ltd., Chatham Street, Reading, Berks RG1 7HT. Tel. Reading 595835. A special service providing most appliances and aids made by manufacturers, with an advice service.

W.B. Pharmaceuticals Ltd., Box 23, Bracknell, Berkshire RG12 4YS. Tel. Bracknell 50222. *Celevac* tablets and granules.

INDEX